MW00747974

Schizophrenia
Breaking Down the Barriers

This publication was supported by an educational grant from

Zeneca Pharma Inc.

Schizophrenia

Breaking Down the Barriers

Edited by

S.G. Holliday, R.J. Ancill and G.W. MacEwan
Department of Psychiatry, St. Vincent's Hospital, Vancouver,
British Columbia, Canada

JOHN WILEY & SONS
Chichester · New York · Brisbane · Toronto · Singapore

Copyright © 1996 by John Wiley & Sons Ltd,
        Baffins Lane, Chichester,
        West Sussex PO19 1UD, England

        National   01243 779777
        International (+44) 1243 779777
        e-mail (for orders and customer service enquiries): cs-books@wiley.co.uk
        Visit our Home Page on http://www.wiley.co.uk
                or http://www.wiley.com

All Rights Reserved. No part of this book may be reproduced, stored in a retrieval
system, or transmitted, in any form or by any means, electronic, mechanical, photocopying,
recording or otherwise, except under the terms of the Copyright, Designs and Patents Act
1988 or under the terms of a licence issued by the Copyright Licensing Agency, 90
Tottenham Court Road, London, UK W1P 9HE, without the permission in writing of the
publisher.

Other Wiley Editorial Offices

John Wiley & Sons, Inc., 605 Third Avenue,
New York, NY 10158-0012, USA

Jacaranda Wiley Ltd, 33 Park Road, Milton,
Queensland 4064, Australia

John Wiley & Sons (Canada) Ltd, 22 Worcester Road,
Rexdale, Ontario M9W 1L1, Canada

John Wiley & Sons (Asia) Pte Ltd, 2 Clementi Loop #02-01,
Jin Xing Distripark, Singapore 0512

British Library Cataloguing in Publication Data

A catalogue record for this book is available from the British Library

ISBN 0-471-967033

Produced from camera ready copy supplied by the editors
Printed and bound in Great Britain by Bookcraft (Bath) Ltd, Midsomer Norton, Somerset
This book is printed on acid-free paper responsibly manufactured from sustainable forestation,
for which at least two trees are planted for each one used for paper production.

Contents

Contributors

Raymond J. Ancill, M.A., M.B., MRCPysch (UK), FRCPC

Head, Department of Psychiatry, St. Vincent's Hospital and Clinical Professor, Department of Psychiatry, University of British Columbia, Vancouver, British Columbia, Canada

Lisa A. Arvanitis, M.D.

Senior Director, CNS, Clinical Research Zeneca Pharmaceuticals, Wilmington, Delaware, United States

P. Asherson,

Department of Psychological Medicine, Institute of Psychiatry, De Crespigny Park, London, United Kingdon

Leona L. Bachrach, Ph.D.

Research Professor of Psychiatry, Maryland Psychiatric Research Center, University of Maryland School of Medicine, Baltimore, Maryland, United States

D. Castle

Department of Psychological Medicine, Institute of Psychiatry, De Crespigny Park, London, United Kingdom

A. Clements

Department of Psychological Medicine, Institute of Psychiatry, De Crespigny Park, London, United Kingdom

Sean W. Flynn, M.D., FRCPC

Fellow, Medical Research Council of Canada, Department of Psychiatry, University of British Columbia, Jack Bell Research Centre, Vancouver, British Columbia, Canada

M. Gill

Department of Psychological Medicine, Institute of Psychiatry, De Crespigny Park, London, United Kingdom

Jeffrey Goldstein, Ph.D.

Principal Pharmacologist, Assistant Director, CNS, Clinical Research Zeneca Pharmaceuticals, Wilmington, Delaware, United States

Hisham Hafez

Courtenay M. Harding, Ph.D.

Assistant Professor of Psychiatry and Associate Director, Program for Public Psychiatry, School of Medicine, University of Colorado, Denver, Colorado, United States

Stephen G. Holliday, Ph.D.

Assistant Head, Department of Psychiatry, St. Vincent's Hospital, Vancouver, British Columbia, Canada

Joel J. Jeffries, M.B. FRCPC

Associate Professor of Psychiatry and Pharmacy, University of Toronto, Staff Psychiatrist, Clarke Institute, Toronto, Ontario, Canada

Barry D. Jones, M.D., FRCPC

Associate Vice President, Research and Development, Eli Lilly Canada, Scarborough, Ontario, Canada

Malcolm Lader, D.Sc., Ph.D., M.D., F.R.C.Psych

Professor of Clinical Psychopharmacology, Institute of Psychiatry, De Crespigny Park, London, United Kingdom

Paul B. Lieberman

G.W. MacEwan, M.D., FRCPC

Director, Adult Psychiatric Services, St. Vincent's Hospital, and Clinical Assistant Professor, Department of Psychiatry, University of British Columbia, Vancouver, British Columbia, Canada

P. McGuffin

Department of Psychological Medicine, University of Wales, College of Medicine, Cardiff, Wales, United Kingdom

Robin M. Murray, DSC, FRCPsych.

Professor and Chairman, Department of Psychological Medicine, Institute of Psychiatry and King's College Hospital, De Crespigny Park, London, United Kingdom

Robert J. Nielsen, M.B.

Clinical Trainee, Department of Psychiatry, St. Vincent's Hospital, Vancouver, British Columbia, Canada

M. Owen

Department of Psychological Medicine, University of Wales, College of Medicine, Cardiff, Wales, United Kingdom

M. Sargeant

Department of Psychological Medicine, University of Wales, College of Medicine, Cardiff, Wales, United Kingdom

Nathan Schaeffer, M.D., FRCPC

Staff Psychiatrist, St. Paul's Hospital, Vancouver, British Columbia, Canada

P. Sham

Department of Psychological Medicine, Institute of Psychiatry, De Crespigny Park, London, United Kingdom

L. james Sheldon, M.D., FRCPC

Director of Consultation Liaison Services, Department of Geriatric Psychiatry, St. Vincent's Hospital, Vancouver, British Columbia, Canada

John S. Strauss

John A. Talbot, M.D.

Professor and Chairman, Department of Psychiatry, University of Maryland, Baltimore, Maryland, United States

C. Taylor

Department of Psychological Medicine, Institute of Psychiatry, De Crespigny Park, London, United Kingdom

C. Walsh

Department of Psychological Medicine, Institute of Psychiatry, De Crespigny Park, London, United Kingdom

D. Watt

Formerly of St. John's Hospital, Stone, Aylesbury, Buckinghamshire, United Kingdom

J. Williams

Department of Psychological Medicine, University of Wales, College of Medicine, Cardiff, Wales, United Kingdom

Preface

This book is a companion piece to Schizophrenia 1996: Breaking Down the Barriers, the fourth in a continuing series of international conferences focusing on the clinical aspects of schizophrenia. The first conference, held in 1990, was titled "Poised for Discovery." And in 1990 many of us felt that we were indeed poised for discovery. The successful introduction of clozapine seemed to herald a new era of pharmacological management of schizophrenia. There was a sense of optimism that genetic research would provide us with a new understanding of the causes of schizophrenia. Epidemiological studies of risk factors also seemed to hold hope for identifying the variables that precipitate schizophrenia. Psychosocial rehabilitation was also emerging as a viable adjunct treatment, with longitudinal studies demonstrating improved outcome following even simple interventions.

The theme of the 1992 conference was "Poised for Change." Looking back at that conference there was a sense that we were moving forward and that the development of novel antipsychotic agents, the expansion of rehabilitation, and the expansion of case-management and individualized treatment approaches would change the way we managed the course of schizophrenic illness. The opening lecture at that conference focused on the strengths and limitations of biological therapies and there were numerous sessions focusing on ways in which novel, supportive environments could help the person with schizophrenia once conventional antipsychotic agents had dealt with acute psychosis.

In 1994, the conference was titled "Exploring the Spectrum of Psychosis." The topic reflected a concern in the field of schizophrenia treatment that we should be taking a broader view of psychosis. The opening lecture in 1994 focused on neural developmental process and discussed how development gone awry could lead to the constellation of schizophrenic symptoms. There was less of a sense of excitement at this conference and more of a concern over getting our therapeutic and management strategies in order. This concern with 'housekeeping' matters probably reflected the fact that neither research, theoretical, or therapeutic breakthroughs were on the horizon.

While trying to find a theme for the 1996 conference, I was struck that many of the problems identified in 1988 when we were developing the 1990 conference remained central in 1996. I was also struck by the number of colleagues an persons with schizophrenia who continued to describe their experience as bein akin to continually running into walls: Therapeutic walls. Economic walls. Wall of Ignorance. Walls of Prejudice. It is clear that neither health car professionals, nor the clients with whom they work have an easy path. The them "Breaking Down the Barrier" is the closest that the organizing committee coul come to capturing that sentiment in a meeting.

The chapters in this book speak to a wide range of barriers. Dr. John Talbot whose thoughtful chapter leads off this book is no stranger to the topic o barriers. As you will see in his chapter, he periodically returns to this topic. hope you will find, as I did, that his longer perspective provides some validatio for our hope that we at least sometimes move in the right direction. Drs. Leon Bachrach and Joel Jeffries discuss an issue that I feel is particularly important the barrier between health care professionals and patients. Starting fror opposite sides of the field - Dr. Bachrach from the patient-authored literature an Dr. Jeffries from the doctor's desk - they manage to wind their way to a interesting middle ground based on the need for mutual recognition and respec between clients and service providers.

Some barriers should be obvious yet somehow manage to escape our attentio until a thoughtful review highlights them. This is clearly the case with Dr Harding's discussion of work. Her analysis reflects a theme that man chronically ill people feel is centrally important: The need to be productive contributing members of society. It is no coincidence that a group of Canadia mental health consumers, when asked to develop a position paper on their long term therapeutic requirements, developed a position paper entitled "A Right t Work - A Need to Work." I cannot help but agree that this barrier may b central to the success or failure of many recovering persons with schizophrenia.

The chapter by Dr. Murray and colleagues reminds us that clear, logical thought when harnessed to sound research strategies, is the best way to overcom barriers to understanding. His chapter is an excellent example of how a questio can be systematically formulate, researched, and answered. The work describe in the chapter clearly contributes to our knowledge of the etiology o schizophrenia. It also stands as an excellent example of how clinical data base can be effectively linked and then used to answer basic research questions.
The chapter by Dr. Sheldon focuses on phenomenology - a time honoure technique that has never quite taken hold in North America. Although th chapter is wide-ranging, the thrust of the argument is that diagnostic technique should be based on a sound investigation of the illness under consideration. A he argues throughout the chapter, failure to develop a clear picture of the natura

ourse of schizophrenia, inevitably leads to an insurmountable barrier - diagnostic confusion.

Dr. Jones and I tried on a very large pair of boots when we developed the chapter on ethical issues surrounding the use of antipsychotic agents. Although, they may have been a bit too large for us, we have done our best to explicate a problem that has bothered both of us for some time - the relative indifference of health care systems to therapeutic advances that could improve the lives of people with schizophrenia. Although the chapter focuses on medication issues, the general argument that society undervalues person's with schizophrenia and, consequently moves slowly, if at all, to implement sound treatment strategies, could be applied to any aspect of treatment and rehabilitation.

Throughout this book one author after another identifies the barrier of treatment resistance as presenting a major problem to the health care system. The chapter by Dr. MacEwan and colleagues describes a systematic approach to diagnosing and treating treatment-resistant schizophrenia. The procedures described in the chapter, and the clinical algorithm for diagnoses and treatment are applicable in most hospital settings.

The chapters by Dr. Goldstein, Dr. Arvenitis, and Dr. Ancill deal with therapeutics, following on the heels of Dr. Jones and my foray into the ethics of antipsychotic use, will clearly survive any heat raised by our discussion. The development of new medication is a necessary part of our overall management of schizophrenia. Data that is offered to support new medications should, in my opinion, be exposed to the highest degree of public scrutiny. I am pleased that we can offer this information to practitioners and researchers alike. Likewise, any attempt to break down the barriers that prevent us from extending therapeutic options to special groups - such as the elderly - should be encouraged. In that regard, Dr. Ancill's chapter is a positive step that moves us towards a more comprehensive view of psychosis across the lifespan.

Editing this book has been a pleasure. Not only were the authors cooperative about deadlines (Dr. Jones and myself excluded), they were to a person enthusiastic about the task. I hope that their enthusiasm and levels of accomplishment will translate into an equally pleasurable experience for the reader.

Stephen G. Holliday
Chairman, Schizophrenia 1996 Conference

BARRIERS TO CARE

John A. Talbott

INTRODUCTION

The topic of this volume, "Breaking Down the Barriers," is an incredibly important one and one which I feel compelled to revisit every ten years or so (Talbott 1978, Bachrach, Talbott & Meyerson 1986). At this point, we have conducted an impressive amount of scientific investigation into the causes and treatment of schizophrenia (Judd 1986) as well as gained a vast amount of experience applying innovative programs to treat those who suffer from this devastating illness (Talbott 1994a). Despite all this, however, we are hardly in a position to state that we can adequately recognize, treat, care and rehabilitate those who suffer from the disease.

First and foremost, we do not have either an adequate knowledge base to enable us to prevent the occurrence of schizophrenia or the technology to adequately treat it or to prevent its recurrence. Disappointingly, in addition to these absolute deficiencies in knowledge, we do not even *fully* utilize those elements of treatment, care and rehabilitation that we *do* know to work (Talbott 1987).

We all know there are barriers to the care of our patients, clients and loved ones, but there is relatively little written about what they are and how we can overcome them (Meyerson 1978, Paul 1978, Meyerson 1987, Talbott 1987) compared to the magnitude of the problem. Indeed, the only book that uses the word *barriers* in its title was published fully a decade ago (Meyerson 1986) and the only book chapter was published nearly a decade before that (Meyerson 1978); the only paper whose title involves "*breaking down barriers*" was also

Schizophrenia: Breaking Down the Barriers. Edited by S.G. Holliday, R.J. Ancill and G.W. MacEwan. © 1996 John Wiley & Sons Ltd

published a decade ago (Reali 1986). Finally, only one contribution specifically compares responses of consumers to those of professionals about the barriers faced (Lynch and Kruzich, 1986).

REVIEW OF THE LITERATURE

The authors of the literature on the barriers to care represent a veritable "who's who" in our field. They address a myriad of such obstacles, specifically financial/economic (Boyer 1987, Gilman & Diamond 1985, Knapp 1990, Levine, Lezak & Diamond 1986, Mueller and Hopp 1987, Rubin 1990, 1990b, Sharfstein 1991, Torrey 1990), attitudinal (Belcher 1988, Gilman & Diamond 1985, Hatfield 1987a, Minkoff 1987, Mueller & Hopp 1987), administrative (Hatfield 1987b, Levine, Lezak & Goldman 1986, Mueller 1987, Yellowlees 1990), legal (Francell, Conn & Gray 1988, Klein 1978, Mueller & Hopp 1987) regulatory (Bachrach 1984, Boyer 1987), bureaucratic (Gilman & Diamond 1985, Talbott 1983) and organizational (Boyer 1987, Corrigan 1995) ones. In addition, other contributions deal with discipline training and practice (Hatfield 1987b, Cooper 1990), collaboration between providers and families (Bernheim 1990, Johnson 1987), service barriers (Grusky 1995), and the bias toward institutional rather than community care (Rubin 1990). Not surprisingly, Leona Bachrach is a major contributor to this corpus, speaking to the barriers to admission, failure to understand the illness, extent of service needs, conflicts in geographic jurisdiction, inappropriate expectation of service planners and providers and homelessness as well as gender, societal and psychological obstacles (Bachrach 1984, 1987a, 1987b, 1990).

As I grappled with the challenge of presenting this overview, I felt caught between two extremes in thinking about the barriers we face; feeling on the one hand, that we merely had to overcome two major barriers — stigma and science — to solve the problem and, on the other hand, that there were too many obstacles in our way to even think of overcoming them.

Therefore, to avoid over-simplifying or over-complicating the number of barriers we face, I did as I have done in the past (Talbott 1994a, Talbott 1994b); that is, I asked experts in the field to help me conceptualize the issue. I asked over a hundred (133) experts in research, service and education in the United States and Canada what they considered to be the top ten barriers. These are people many of whose names you would recognize, some of whom are represented in this volume; among them scientists, practitioners, advocates, family members, and patients or ex-patients. Since I received only 52 answers, a

39% response rate, this is hardly a scientific study, but I believe it served its goal of providing the full range of the obstacles that I desired.

In this overview, I will present a compilation of some of the over 200 barriers my respondents mentioned that we currently face, provide you with the top twenty, highlight some of the ones I found most interesting and conclude by addressing how these many barriers must be overcome.

BARRIERS

In the following discussion, items presented in **bold** type represent major barriers cited by respondents.

The *illness, schizophrenia, itself* was one of the most important issues mentioned by my respondents. First came the barrier of our **lack of understanding of the disease,** its mechanisms, etiology, pathophysiology, biologic underpinnings, etc.

Second mentioned were the **symptoms, impairment and disability** that result from schizophrenia that often cause the sufferer to be unable to seek or comply with treatment. Included in these are the sufferer's lack of insight and judgment; negative symptoms, poor motivation, social withdrawal and apathy; denial of illness; paranoia, delusional ideas and disorganization; chronicity and/or recurrence; ego deficits which often lead to a poor knowledge of services and the state of poverty that often results; interference with psychosocial rehabilitation, which is made difficult because of the modality's reliance on personal relationships; and poor job skills.

Cited third was **co-morbidity**. This involves both the presence in sufferers of schizophrenia of alcohol and/or drug abuse as well as the secondary depression or demoralization that often accompanies the illness.

Treatment issues were also frequently mentioned. Largely, these were problems associated with **medication**, specifically: intolerance to its side effects leading to non-compliance; not having more effective medications; patients' non-continuance on maintenance medications; restricted formularies; patients' resistance to depot medications; the lack of a simple urine test to assess levels of compliance; and misuse followed by "non-compliance."

Other treatment and prevention issues include the fact, mentioned earlier, that we still have no definitive treatment for the illness nor ability to prevent it.

Systems issues were also frequently cited, although they may refer much more to the American non-system of care than would be true in Canada or Europe. Most mentioned here were our **fragmented and poorly-coordinated treatment**, care, housing and support systems, especially in the community, resulting in our inability to provide integrated and/or comprehensive services and lack of a centralized authority as well as our inability to effect good coordination between inpatient and community services.

Along with this overarching problem were: the **lack of continuity of care** as well as poor continuity of persons necessary to prevent relapse; the lack of **structure and support**, including housing; the paucity of **case managers** or continuity agents for all patients; and the absence of integration of medication management and other therapies.

Service deficiencies were also commonly cited, such as too **little focus on rehabilitation**; **restrictive admission policies** of community programs (to exclude all but "motivated patients"); inaccessible, **geographically distant services**; excessively brief hospitalization policies; criminalization of the mentally ill, e.g., overuse of jails as alternative treatment resources; the lack of connections with primary care; the lack of integration of psychiatric and addictions treatment along with a lack of treatment programs for the dually diagnosed.

Several issues are specific to the United States; for example, the fact that the disability secondary to the illness leads to care in the public sector with its politicization and bureaucratization; the problem posed from the fact that the treatment of the schizophrenia is complicated, necessitating the involvement of multiple providers; the issue that there are no real systems of care in the United States permitting easy access to care; the failure to link funding streams to patients; the lack of insurance structures in the United States, like capitation, that would create incentives for preventive approaches, etc.; the difficulty gaining access to a complicated system; the difficulty gaining access to entitlements; the absence of a national health care policy; and the failure to develop well-articulated national standards of what is appropriate care, what is and is not effective and what should and should not be reimbursed.

Then there are the barriers posed by the lack of available resources, e.g., an inadequate array of accessible resources (numbers and funding), including: **mental health resources,** such as inadequate effective community treatment resources, especially outreach, home care and mobile treatment; inadequate numbers of psychosocial rehabilitation programs, especially ones providing long-term rehabilitation; inadequate hospital beds for those needing intermediate and long-term stays; inadequate hospital beds for those needing acute care; inadequate numbers of services for the dually diagnosed; long waiting lists in outpatient clinics; an absence of crisis intervention during relapses; and inadequate residential treatment services. The respondents also mentioned inadequate **non-mental health resources**, such as inadequate affordable and appropriate housing with appropriate levels of supervision; inadequate public and other transportation; inadequate transitional and mainstream employment; inadequate meeting of patients' basic needs; inadequate access to physical care; and inadequate support networks and safe havens.

In addition, my respondents, who it should be remembered were in large part from the United States, commented on problems in *inadequate funding and reimbursement*, including inadequate funding and/or reimbursement of services, such as extended (long-term) care, e.g., asylum; structured psychosocial rehabilitation programs; funding for anything but medication; alternatives to hospitals and emergency rooms, e.g., respite care and crisis care; outreach; and even treatment itself.

In addition, they commented on **our funding and reimbursement complexities**, especially in our public entitlements, e.g., Medicaid and Medicare; the fragmentation in the funding of what patients need; the lack of adequate income support and other benefits, as well as disincentives in our social security system that discourage patients from working; and the lack of research on and attempts to prevent the high cost of care. They also noted the **high cost** of treatment to patients/families, especially for our newer medications and the financial barriers to providing proper treatment, e.g., our history of providing financial incentives for hospitalization and psychotherapy rather than psychosocial interventions. In addition, in the United States, many citizens still have **poor or no insurance** or other reimbursement (if they do, there is a lack of parity and the presence of discrimination in most policies); our public system has been affected by Medicaid cuts and there have been reductions in the funding of public programs and conversion of public facilities to a managed care format.

Finally, in the area of reimbursement, they commented on the current problems with **managed care**, which maintains it is interested in "managing care" to improve quality as much as controlling or cutting costs, but in fact appears quite different, frustrating care-givers with denial of payments, limitations on lengths of stay and models that mitigate against long-term care, wrap-around services, rehabilitation and consumer-operated services.

Many items related to barriers posed by *society, the public and politicians*. Not surprisingly, the most common of these was **stigma** (e.g., prejudice or bias based on fear of illness, violence, or contagion) but also the lack of social status and political advocacy for patients and the lack of interest and the lack of awareness (e.g., ignorance) of both the condition itself and treatment efficacy. Given this, it is not surprising that they thought that a major problem was the reluctance of politicians to adequately fund state services and the prevailing current conservative political philosophy in the United States.

Several persons mentioned barriers posed by **public attitudes, values**, etc., for instance: our values on autonomy and independence rather than interdependence; our attitude of sometimes "blaming the victim;" our frequent "NIMBY" (not in my backyard) residential constraints; the negative attitudes generated by the visibility of the homeless and the opposition of some religious sects. Others commented that there was no place in the social fabric for persons suffering from schizophrenia and that we were facing acceleration in community disintegration, including dangerous streets, crime and homelessness.

Professional issues were often cited. Continuing a longstanding concern about clinicians, at least in the United States, the respondents cited: the lack of **interest in, rewards for and commitment toward** the treatment of serious mental illness as well as a lack of willingness to treat those who are angry, violent, unpredictable, unattractive, drug-abusing, and have a poor prognosis or are on Medicaid. They also cited some **negative professional attitudes**, including: negativity about treatability and the expectation for cure; a reluctance to make the diagnosis of schizophrenia; an unwillingness on the part of physicians to do "medication checks" without overall responsibility for the patient; passivity; intolerance of "differentness" and treating patients as if they had a neuroleptic deficiency disease, not a biopsychosocial one.

The respondents commented that one barrier was the paucity of **adequately trained professionals,** citing poor training and education, including continuing education, especially regarding medication, psychosocial rehabilitation and psychoeducation and commented that too much care was provided by inexperienced, uncaring or ignorant practitioners. Several commented on issues of **clinical competence**, such as the difficulty of correctly making a diagnosis without a laboratory test; not using proven effective care (such as assertive and family treatment); the failure to combine modalities; being unaware of the illness; and a poor understanding of how to deal with schizophrenia.

Others were more sympathetic, stating that many professionals were overworked and that working with patients suffering from schizophrenia was truly time-consuming. Several comments related to the negative effect of rotating psychiatrists in community mental health centers; the fact that too few psychiatrists have admitting privileges in hospitals and that there needed to be more collaboration between professionals and consumers and family groups.

Patient issues included barriers posed by: patients' lack of knowledge of services; their negative attitude toward services; their fear of becoming to dependent on services; their "uncooperativeness" and their frequent inability to provide feedback to professionals.

Family issues included: the lack of family and family support, denial of illness in their relatives or lack of awareness of illness and/or treatment; and inadequate support for care-givers, such as the lack of respite care.

Issues involving both patients and families were: the "non-compliance" of patients and family; a reluctance to use existing care; a lack of confidence in professionals and services; and the lack of education of patients and families about symptoms, services, and medications.

Legal constraints centered around the barriers to involuntary commitment, and respondents favored: easier involuntary inpatient commitment; easier involuntary outpatient commitment; easing the social legislation limiting hospitalization and treatment measures; enabling others to control patients' welfare and disability benefits; and the cumbersome legal system in the United States.

Demographic/cultural issues that were felt to be barriers included: socioeconomic status (e.g., poverty); race; ethnicity; and age. Some of the barriers were felt to actually stem from prejudicial "'isms:" e.g., racism; sexism; "classism" and other forms of prejudice.

Research issues included not enough funding to test hypotheses; slow biomedical research progress; slow research dissemination; insufficient knowledge on how to help the population with work and loneliness; inadequate research on issues such as whether American health maintenance organizations (HMOs) can care for such patients; and NARSAD's over-emphasis on biological research.

Public education barriers were: the lack of large numbers of recovered patients as examples of good treatment; and the lack of public education about services.

Professional educational barriers mentioned were: the lack of an "integrative theory," in part because of our fragmented clinical orientations (rehabilitation, clinical, social support emphases, coming from different and separate clinicians); our failure to achieve effective interdisciplinary teams; and our use of imprecise, irrelevant service delivery concepts.

RANK ORDER

The barriers most commonly mentioned by respondents are presented in Table 1 in rank order.

Table 1. Most Commonly Mentioned Barriers

Stigma (32)
Fragmentation and poor-coordination (18)
Intolerance to side effects—non-compliance (14)
Inadequate housing (13)
Lack of interest, rewards and commitment (12)
Poor training and education (12)
Alcohol/drugs (11)
Cost of treatment, especially newer medications (10)
Inadequate funding/reimbursement of care (10)
Lack of more effective medications (10)
Inadequate array of accessible resources (10)
Lack of understanding of the illness (9)
Resultant symptoms—treatment (8)
Lack of insight and judgment (7)

DISCUSSION

My discussion will concentrate on what I found interesting in the responses I received to my unscientific survey and then, in the following section, I will discuss how we can use this list of barriers to break them down. In looking over the compilation, I was struck by five items in particular.

Most striking to me was the juxtaposition of the large number of persons noting the power of the illness itself and its resultant symptoms, impairment and disability, with the much smaller number of persons mentioning lack of definitive treatment for it as a barrier. Instead, respondents commented on the lack of more effective medication. Is this a reflection of our view that only medication will solve the problem, rather than prevention and psychosocial approaches or that, on the other hand, everyone takes for granted the fact that we have no definitive treatment?

Second, I was struck by the small number of persons who thought that working with persons suffering from schizophrenia is time-consuming, exhausting work; a major obstacle cited by Paul in 1978. Is this because we've finally educated and interested an adequate number of professionals to treat persons suffering from schizophrenia who actually see this element as part of their work, rather than as an annoying add-on to what they would really like to be doing, or because stating that it is tough work is politically incorrect?

Third, the response that research has not focused enough on the very real but everyday problems of work and loneliness struck a poignant note with me. I realize research and researchers cannot be directed, but is there a way to encourage research into the practical obstacles faced by all our patients suffering from schizophrenia?

Fourth, I was disappointed by the response that our public systems of care have so failed our patients, in part due to over-politicization and over-bureaucratization, despite all that has been written and spoken about system deficiencies (Talbott 1978, Bachrach 1987, Hatfield 1987, Meyerson 1987). I suppose that any systematic attempt to solve any problem brings with it politics and bureaucracy, but it is a shame that political needs take precedence over human needs. I'm reminded of a statement made a few years ago by the head of the union representing the employees in the New York City hospital system that it was not a health system but an employment one. Can we not have a better balance between political and patient needs?

Fifth, despite all that has been written and advocated over the last 40 years since deinstitutionalization began about the need for more alternatives to hospitals, easier access to care, more psychosocial rehabilitation and case management for every person suffering from schizophrenia, etc. (Talbott 1980), adequate resources and systems are simply not there.

I would also like to comment on the survey itself. I did not separate consumers', providers' and administrators' responses and thus saw nothing like the division Lynch & Krusich (1986) did, where professionals attributed primary responsibility for barriers to "client resistance" while consumers identified the primary problem as a financial one. Also, I was struck by the range of responses, the care and compassion revealed in the comments and the grasp of the scope of the problem that my respondents had. They and their patients may face large barriers to care, but as I read their responses they appear realistically critical but not necessarily discouraged.

Finally, with such a diverse literature in the subject, it is hard to know how representative this list of barriers is. However, compared to Paul's (1978),

Meyerson's (1978, 1987) and Bachrach's (Bachrach 1984, 1987a, 1987b, 1990) publications, I am struck with the similarities. All three organized their barriers somewhat differently: Paul (1978) into categories of obstacles in Prevailing Attitudes and Beliefs; Legal and Ethical Regulation; Bureaucratic, Administrative and Political Obstacles; and Technical-Methodological ones: and Meyerson (1987) separates those pertaining to professionals, patients, care systems, financing and the law. But Meyerson (1978) clearly identifies stigma as enemy number one, as have my respondents 20 years later. Naturally items such as managed care were not present in these earlier contributions. However, in general there is great concordance; leading either to the pessimistic conclusion that we haven't done much to eliminate the barriers to care in the past few decades or the optimistic one that we now have a clearer idea of what we and our patients are up against.

BREAKING DOWN THE BARRIERS

With the presence of so many barriers to the care and treatment of persons suffering from schizophrenia, it is clear that no single, simple solution is conceivable. Instead, concerted efforts in several areas are called for. These include research and service initiatives for the benefit of those who suffer from this disorder, as well as educational ones directed toward society, politicians, professionals, families and consumers.

Research remains a high priority, but as my respondents have suggested, it should be targeted not only toward pharmacological interventions but at total prevention of the illness and elimination of all its symptoms, impairment and disability. This should include such everyday problems as work and loneliness. I would add as well, that since we have failed so miserably at reducing the stigma of mental illnesses, we need to know much more about what has worked to educate the public about such previously highly stigmatized diseases as tuberculosis and cancer, to more effectively educate the public.

Services remain a critical target for reform. This must include what we have heard preached since deinstitutionalization began in 1955; e.g., the easy access and wide availability of a range of high quality ambulatory and inpatient services that provide all acute, intermittent and long-term treatment, care and rehabilitation needed, as well as community support and case management. The barriers to fulfilling this widely-agreed upon goal also remain as elusive in most parts of the world as does the elimination of the disease or stigma. In addition, added to the barriers that existed in 1955, we now have the complications posed by the almost universal availability of drugs and alcohol.

Especially regarding the American non-system of care, it is clear that the elimination of our fragmented and complex administrative and financing mechanisms is as important as resource provision. How much of this "American disease" will be helped or aggravated for those suffering from schizophrenia in the next few years, given our past decades' romance with one way of "managing care," remains to be seen.

Finally, there is the huge area of education. This includes education of the public and politicians about the disease, its treatability, the consequences of its not being treated, e.g., devastating symptoms, profound disability and severe impairment leading to ruination of lives, devastation of families, loss of job skills, poverty and the inability to manage everyday tasks all citizens take for granted. It also must include the effort to educate all citizens about the balance between societal and individual rights.

But as importantly, we need to educate professionals in diagnosis, modern effective treatment and rehabilitation; about dealing with not only schizophrenia itself but co-occurring substance abuse, depression and demoralization. Needed as well is a concerted effort to continue encouraging those who wish to work with the most seriously ill in our society to do so and re-education of those who do not, as to their responsibilities as professionals to care for all in need.

While this may seem like an awesome list of barriers and even more awesome list of efforts to break them down, it goes without saying that knowledge must precede action if it is to be effective. Unfortunately, too often in the past we have cried out in the dark without knowing what we were facing; I hope now we can finally appreciate all the barriers that face us, crack them into manageable bits and slowly but surely break them down.

SUMMARY

This chapter constitutes a beginning of a much broader discussion to be presented in this volume; that is, of breaking down all the barriers to adequate care, treatment and rehabilitation of those suffering from schizophrenia. I began by summarizing the barriers provided by a sample of experts on the disorder, including scientists, practitioners, family members and consumers or former consumers. I then discussed five interesting issues that emerged, followed by a discussion of how we could address breaking down the barriers. I conclude that it is only by realistically understanding and assessing the barriers that face us, that we can finally break them down.

REFERENCES

Bachrach, L.L. (1984) "Research on Services for the Homeless Mentally Ill", *Hospital and Community Psychiatry*, 35(9), 910–913.

Bachrach, L.L., Talbott, J.A. and Meyerson, A.T. (1986) "The Chronic Psychiatric Patient as a 'Difficult' Patient: A Conceptual Analysis". In *Barriers to Treating the Chronic Mentally Ill. New Directions for Mental Health Services* (Ed. A.T. Meyerson), No. 33, Jossey-Bass, San Francisco, CA, 35–49.

Bachrach, L.L. (1986) "The Homeless Mentally Ill in the General Hospital: A Question of Fit", *General Hospital Psychiatry*, 8(5), 340–349.

Bachrach, L.L. (1987a) "Issues in Identifying and Treating the Homeless Mentally Ill", *New Directions for Mental Health Services*, 35, 43–62.

Bachrach, L.L. (1987b) "Deinstitutionalization in the United States: Promises and Prospects", *New Directions for Mental Health Services*, 35, 75–90.

Bachrach, L.L. (1990) "Homeless Mentally Ill Women: A Special Population", In *Women's Progress: Promises and problems. Women in Context: Development and Stresses* (Eds. J. Spurlock and C.B. Robinowitz), Plenum Press, New York, 189–201.

Belcher, J.R. and First, R.J. (1987) "The Homeless Mentally Ill: Barriers to Effective Service Delivery", *Journal of Applied Social Sciences*, 12(1), 62–78.

Bernheim, K.F. (1990) "Principles of Professional and Family Collaborations", *Hospital and Community Psychiatry*, 41(12), 1353-1355.

Boyer, C.A. (1987) "Obstacles in Urban Housing Policy for the Chronically Mentally Ill", *New Directions for Mental Health Services* (Ed. D. Mechanics), Jossey-Bass, San Francisco, CA, 36:71–81.

Cohen, N.L. (1991) *Psychiatric Outreach to the Mentally Ill,* Jossey-Bass, San Francisco, CA.

Cooper, J.E. (1990) "Professional Obstacles to Implementation and Diffusion of Innovative Approaches to Mental Health Care". In *Mental Health Care Delivery: Innovations, Impediments and Implementation* (Eds. I.M. Marks and R.A. Scott), Cambridge University Press, Cambridge, England, 233–253.

Corrigan, P.W. (1995) "Wanted: Champions of Psychiatric Rehabilitation", *American Psychologist*, 50(7), 514–521.

Cutler, D.L. (1986) "Community Residential Options for the Chronically Mentally Ill", *Community Mental Health Journal*, 22(1), 61–73.

Dencker, S.J. and Liberman, R.P. (1995) "From Compliance to Collaboration in the Treatment of Schizophrenia", *International Clinical Psychopharmacology*, 9(5), 75–78.

Dennis, D.L., Buckner, J.C., Lipton, F.R. and Levine, I.S. (1991) "A Decade of Research and Services for Homeless Mentally Ill Persons: Where Do We Stand?", *American Psychologist*, 46(11), 1129–1138.

Dill, A.E. and Rochefort, D.A. (1989) "Coordination, Continuity and Centralized Control: A Policy Perspective on Service Strategies for the Chronic Mentally Ill", *Journal of Social Issues*, 45(3), 145–159.

France L, C.G., Conn, V.S. and Gray, D.P. (1988) "Families' Perceptions of Burden of Care for Chronic Mentally Ill Relatives", *Hospital & Community Psychiatry*, 39(12), 1296–1300.

Gilman, S.R. and Diamond, R.J. (1985) "Economic Analysis in Community Treatment of the Chronically Mentally Ill", *New Directions for Mental Health Services*, 26, 77–84.

Grusky, O. (1995) "The Organization and Effectiveness of Community Mental Health Systems", *Administration and Policy in Mental Health*, 22(4), 361–388.

Hatfield, A.B. (1986) "Systems Resistance to Effective Family Coping", In *Barriers to Treating the Chronic Mentally Ill. New Directions for Mental Health Services* (Ed. A.T. Meyerson), No. 33, Jossey-Bass, San Francisco, CA, 51–62.

Hatfield, A.B. (1987a) "Consumer Issues in Mental Illness", *New Directions for Mental Health Services*, 34, 35–42.

Hatfield, A.B. (1987b) "Systems Resistance to Effective Family Coping", *New Directions for Mental Health Services*, 33, 51–62

Jahiel, R.I. (1992) "Homelessness: A Prevention-Oriented Approach". In *New School for Social Research, Graduate School of Management and Policy, Health Services Management and Policy Program, Adjunct Professor of Health Services Research and Policy*. Johns Hopkins Press, Baltimore, MD.

Judd, L.L. (1986) "The Future of the Basic Science of Psychiatry". In *Our Patients' Future in a Changing World* (Ed. J.A. Talbott) American Psychiatric Press Inc., Washington, DC, 11–22.

Johnson, D.L. (1987) "Professional Family Collaboration", *New Directions for Mental Health Services,* 34, 73–79.

Klein, J.I. (1986) "Resistances to Care of the Chronic Patient: A Lawyer's Contribution". In *Barriers to Treating the Chronic Mentally Ill. New Directions for Mental Health Services* (Ed. A.T. Meyerson), No. 33, Jossey-Bass, San Francisco, CA, 87–95.

Knapp, M. (1990) "Economic Barriers to Innovation in Mental Health Care: Community Care in the United Kingdom". In *Mental Health Care Delivery: Innovations, Impediments and Implementation* (Eds. I.M. Marks and R.A. Scott), Cambridge University Press, Cambridge, England, 204–219.

Levine, I.S., Lezak, A.D. and Goldman, H.H. (1986) "Community Support Systems for the Homeless Mentally Ill", *New Directions for Mental Health Services,* 30, 27–42.

Lynch, M.M. and Kruzich, J.M. (1986) "Needs Assessment of the Chronically Mentall Ill: Practitioners and Client Perspectives", *Administration in Mental Health*, 13(4), 237-248.

Marks, I.M. and Scott, R.A. (1990) *Mental Health Care Delivery: Innovations Impediments and Implementation.* Cambridge University Press, Cambridge, England.

Mechanic, D. (1989) "Toward the Year 2000 in U.S. Mental Health Policymaking and Administration". In *Handbook on Mental Health Policy in the United States* (Ed. D.A Rochefort), Greenwood Press, Westport, CT, 477–503.

Meyerson, A.T. (1978) "What Are the Barriers or Obstacles to Treatment and Care of th Chronically Disabled Mentally Ill". In *The Chronic Mental Patient* (Ed. J.A. Talbott American Psychiatric Association, Washington, DC, 128–134.

Meyerson, A.T. and Herman, G.H. (1986) "Systems Resistance to the Chronic Patient" In *Barriers to Treating the Chronic Mentally Ill. New Directions for Mental Healt Services* (Ed. A.T. Meyerson), No. 33, Jossey-Bass, San Francisco, CA, 21–34.

Meyerson, A.T., (1986) *Barriers to Treating the Chronic Mentally Ill. New Direction for Mental Health Services* No. 33, Jossey-Bass, San Francisco, California.

Miller, G.E. (1988) "Role of Psychiatrists in the Public Mental Health System" *Psychiatric Quarterly*, 59(2), 88–102.

Minkoff, K. (1987) "Resistance of Mental Health Professionals to Working with th Chronic Mentally Ill", *New Directions for Mental Health Services*, 33, 3–20.

Minkoff, K. (1986) "Resistance of Mental Health Professionals to Working with th Chronic Mentally Ill". In *Barriers to Treating the Chronic Mentally Ill. New Direction for Mental Health Services* (Ed. A.T. Meyerson), No. 33, Jossey-Bass, San Francisco CA, 3–20.

Mueller, B.J. and Hopp, M. (1986-87) "Attitudinal, Administrative, Legal, and Fisca Barriers to Case Management in Social Rehabilitation of the Mentally Ill", *Internationa Journal of Mental Health*, 15(4), 44–58.

National Academy of Sciences, Institute of Medicine, Committee on Health Care fo Homeless People (1988) *Homelessness,* National Academy Press, Washington, DC.

Paul, G.L. (1978) "The Implementation of Treatment Programs for Chronic Menta Patients: Obstacles and Recommendations". In *The Chronic Mental Patient* (Ed. J.A Talbott), American Psychiatric Association, Washington, DC, 99–133.

Reali, M. (1986) "Breaking Down Barriers: The Work of the Community Mental Healt Services of Trieste in the Prison and Judicial Settings", *International Journal of Law an Psychiatry*, 8(4), 395–412.

Rubin, J. (1990) "Economic Barriers to Implementing Innovative Mental Health Care in the United States". In *Mental Health Care Delivery: Innovations, Impediments and Implementation* (Eds. I.M. Marks and R.A. Scott), Cambridge University Press, Cambridge, England, 220–232.

Sharfstein, S.S. (1986) "Reimbursement Resistance to Treatment and Support for the Long-Term Mental Patient". In *Barriers to Treating the Chronic Mentally Ill. New Directions for Mental Health Services* (Ed. A.T. Meyerson), No. 33, Jossey-Bass, San Francisco, CA, 75–85.

Sharfstein, S.S. (1991) "Prospective Cost Allocations for the Chronic Schizophrenic Patient", *Schizophrenia Bulletin*, 17(3), 395–400.

Talbott, J.A. (1978) *The Chronic Mental Patient*, American Psychiatric Association, Washington, DC.

Talbott, J.A. (1980) "Toward a public policy on the chronic mental patient", *A.J. Orthopsych*, 50, 43–53.

Talbott, J.A. (1983) A Special Population: The Elderly Deinstitutionalized Chronically Mentally Ill Patient", *Psychiatric Quarterly*, 55, 90–105.

Talbott, J.A. (1987) "The Chronic Mentally Ill: What Do We Now Know and Why Aren't We Implementing What We Know". In *The Chronic Mental Patient/II* (Eds. W.W. Menninger and G. Hannah), American Psychiatric Press, Inc., Washington, D.C.

Talbott, J.A. (1994a) "Lessons Learned About the Chronic Mentally Ill Since 1955", In *Schizophrenia 1994: Exploring the Spectrum of Psychosis* (eds. R.J. Ancill, S. Holliday and J. Higenbottam) Wiley, Chichester, 1–20.

Talbott, J.A. (1994b) "Deinstitutionalization, Emergency Services, and the Third Revolution in Mental Health Services in the United States". In *Reflections sur la pratique clinique des urgences psychiatriques* (Eds. S. Lamarre and F. Grunberg). in press.

Torrey, E.F. (1990) "Economic Barriers to Widespread Implementation of Model Programs for the Seriously Mentally Ill", *Hospital and Community Psychiatry*, 41(5), 526–531.

Yellowlees, H. (1990) "Administrative Barriers to Implementation and Diffusion of Innovative Approaches to Mental Health Care in the United Kingdom". In *Mental Health Care Delivery: Innovations, Impediments and Implementation* (Eds. I.M. Marks and R.A. Scott), Cambridge University Press, Cambridge, England, 167–178.

2

WHAT DO PATIENTS SAY ABOUT PROGRAM PLANNING? PERSPECTIVES FROM THE PATIENT-AUTHORED LITERATURE

Leona L. Bachrach

Persons who are or have been patients in the mental health service system have for some years been writing about their experiences as service recipients. They are, perforce, experts in the field of mental health program planning, and their products are often frank, articulate, and exceedingly sensitive. In fact, their writings contain important clues and information from which mental health program planners might take direction; yet surprisingly little note has been taken of the patient-authored literature in the development of program initiatives for mentally ill individuals.

This chapter presents partial findings from an ongoing literature review of patient-authored writings retrieved through a Medline search of periodical literature that was published since 1983. Occasional earlier writings by patients that seem especially relevant to the subject of this inquiry have also been examined, as have patient-authored books and writings from a variety of miscellaneous sources — the so-called "fugitive literature" consisting of letters, newspaper articles, agency publications, conference proceedings, and other unindexed statements.

The chapter's purpose is to establish points of agreement between patient-authors and professionals who design, plan, and implement mental health programs. Are the pet planning concepts that professionals espouse reinforced or

Schizophrenia: Breaking Down the Barriers. Edited by S.G. Holliday, R.J. Ancill and G.W. MacEwan. © 1996 John Wiley & Sons Ltd

contradicted in patients' writings?   And what, if anything, that is important to patient-authors have professionals tended to overlook?

To answer these questions I employ three basic concepts that have assumed increasing popularity in professional program planning circles in recent years: the notion that treatment resistance among patients, sometimes called "difficult patienthood," has more than one source; the notion that the disabilities accompanying severe mental illness are complex and multivariate; and the idea that service planning for mentally ill persons should, ideally, be tailored to the needs of each individual member of the patient population. These three concepts are probably more accurately described as conceptual "fields," for each is intricately intertwined with other established program planning principles and concepts (Bachrach, 1989).

It is important to note at the outset that this chapter does not purport to present a comprehensive review of patient-authored literature; the focus here is limited specifically to program planning and service delivery issues as they are discussed in that literature. Nor is this chapter concerned with the politics of the patient rights movement or with advocacy for mental patients, important as those matters are. Instead, this chapter's aim is to take a small step toward bridging the gap between the perspectives of patient-authors and professional program designers. To say this differently, this chapter represents an effort to assess what outsiders' looking in may learn from insiders' speaking out about issues in mental health program planning and service delivery.

On the assumption that patients' own words are superior to paraphrases, direct quotations are liberally interspersed throughout this review. Serendipitously, this carries a distinct esthetic reward, for patients' writings are often poetic and lyrical, as the late Jack Weinberg (1978) noted when he wrote about "the words of the emotionally ill...the poetry of the anguished mentality." By way of example, a patient at the Rhode Island Institute of Mental Health (1984) who signs his name as Tom writes:

Getting out of here	To see the rain
And into something	When it comes
Like work	But to be able
Or something payable	To hang around and hope
Like caddying	Helps a lot
I've had some good days	But to sit
And some rainy ones	And be incarcerated
Sometimes it would	Almost drives you
Break your heart	To be tapioca

Another patient at the same hospital who signs his name as Robert writes:

> Fill my mind with knowledge
> Fill my body with definition
> Fill my life with total well being
> Fill my pockets with money
> Fill my head with normal thoughts
> Fill my nerves with relaxation
> Fill myself with the old me

PLANNING CONCEPTS

Mental health program planning today—at least on paper if not in actual fact—is greatly influenced by the convergence of three interrelated conceptual developments: first, emerging ideas about what makes a given patient treatment resistant, noncompliant, or "difficult"; second, our understanding of the concept of disability as it affects mentally ill individuals; and, third, our promotion of individualized treatment planning for members of the patient population.

DIFFICULT PATIENTHOOD

The words "difficult patient," which are frequently used to indicate treatment resistance or lack of cooperation (Bachrach, Talbott, and Meyerson, 1987), are inherently both stigmatizing and contradictory, since "all patients who have been designated as having a psychiatric condition are expected to be problems to themselves as well as to their respective environments, which includes the psychiatrist who comes into contact with them" (Chrzanowski, 1980). Nonetheless, this term is in common use in the current literature on program planning where, typically, difficult patienthood is traced to one or more of three interrelated precipitants (Bachrach, Talbott, and Meyerson, 1987).

First, difficult patienthood may be attributed to the patient himself or herself: to certain behaviors, characteristics, or attributes that distinguish that patient from other "non-difficult" patients. Neill (1979) reports that difficult patients tend generally to be more demanding, more puzzling, less likely to evoke empathy, more dangerous to themselves and others, more attention-seeking and manipulative, more likely to polarize staff, more technically difficult as psychiatric cases, and more likely to misuse medication, than non-difficult patients.

Second, difficult patienthood may be attributed to the clinician who works with the patient—or, more specifically, to the clinician's biases, expectations, or "rules" that are superimposed on the clinical interaction. Examples of such unwritten rules would include stipulations that the illness be treatable and preferably curable; that the patient be fully cooperative; and that the patient regard his or her condition as something that must be changed (Jeffrey, 1979). When a patient breaks these or other similar rules, the clinician may well perceive that individual as a difficult patient.

It is exceedingly difficult in practice to separate the first and second sources of difficult patienthood, for a person's characteristics, attributes, and behaviors are only contextually troublesome; and while they may be necessary, they are not sufficient for the definition of difficult patienthood (Bachrach, Talbott, and Meyerson, 1987). A particular patient's behaviors or attributes are thus difficult only when they are perceived to be so by clinicians, administrators, or service planners.

Third, difficult patienthood may be attributed to the service system itself, or more precisely to deficits within that system. When the service system lacks sufficient will or resources to provide continuity of care and comprehensive care, it tends to build a protective shield around itself. Harris and Bergman (1986–87) have introduced the concept of the "narcissistically vulnerable system" to describe the defensive postures assumed by service structures that "are primarily concerned with maintaining an often fragile sense of self-esteem." It is not uncommon for the service system to identify patients whom it will not or cannot serve, or whom it will not or cannot treat, as difficult patients and thereby absolve itself of the obligation to care for these individuals.

These three sources of difficult patienthood are highly interactive and, according to the literature, rarely operate independently (Bachrach, Talbott, and Meyerson, 1987). Conceptually, the most critical point concerning them is that it takes more than just a patient to make a difficult patient. It takes a context as well — a context that consists of both clinician variables and system variables.

PATIENTS' VIEWS

These sources of difficult patienthood are fully acknowledged in the patient-authored literature, often with great insight. As for the first, patient-authored writings frankly admit that patients at times exhibit behaviors or characteristics that are sufficiently removed from the mainstream that they are troublesome to clinicians, service systems, relatives, and society at large. Indeed, the patient-authored literature frequently implies, and sometimes explicitly states, that such behaviors and characteristics should be considered predictable manifestations of severe and invasive illness.

Moreover, patient-authors appear to have an unusual talent for demonstrating the intrinsic interdependence between the first and second sources of difficult patienthood. They frequently observe that patients' troublesome behaviors, attributes, and characteristics must be understood as the "flip-side" of clinicians' attitudes and expectations. Thus, Sharp (1988) implores clinicians to recognize and acknowledge their own role in promoting difficult patienthood: "If you don't like someone, get them a doctor who does like them. Don't just get stonefaced and argumentative, but have the strength to let go. Be more responsive."

Indeed, Sharp (1988), who in her writings often addresses clinicians directly in the second person, is not above mixing a bit of irony and humor with her eloquence:

> Doctors, pills are pills, however you slice them, and you have all the control, but only the patient knows if he wants to take one a second time, whether it helps or hurts. You're not veterinarians, so your patients can speak and you will get your best clues by listening to them, and by believing them you will get the truth.

Blaska (1994) is also concerned that service providers "need major attitudinal changes." She writes:

> Psychiatric staff's primary attitude should not be punitive ("What is she or he doing wrong?") but supportive ("How is he or she hurting?"). Staff must learn not to be afraid of us. Often it is we who are afraid of staff as well as of others.

And Brundage (1983) concludes that:

> The effectiveness in reaching and working with patients rests largely upon the ability of the caregiver to perceive and comprehend how particular patients are experiencing their illnesses...Meticulous honesty and fairness on the part of the caregiver is important. Sometimes patients...get even more confused in the face of ambiguity and deception...Tact and understanding of the patients' distress will go a long way toward increasing self-esteem and feelings of self-worth.

Patient-authors are similarly often direct and persuasive in offering illustrations of the relationship between difficult patienthood and system inadequacy. They frequently report personal histories filled with searches for appropriate and responsive programs—programs that are, most often, simply not to be found. Or, if the programs can be found, the barriers to using them are perceived as multiple, subtle, and generally insuperable. The message here is clear. Patient-authors tell us in no uncertain terms that if patients are to become more compliant and less burdensome to the system of care, the system must do its part to welcome them and respond to their needs.

In fact, concern with system deficits led one well-known patient-author, Priscilla Allen, to formulate a patients' bill of rights in 1974. Allen later served as one of the Commissioners in President Carter's Commission on Mental Health; and her message — that comprehensive services, full access to care, and individualized treatments delivered with regard for patients' personhood and dignity must be made available to mentally ill individuals—is frequently repeated in today's patient-authored literature.

SOURCES OF DISABILITY

A second conceptual field that strongly influences contemporary service planning for mentally ill individuals involves the notion of disability. There is growing awareness today that disability typically derives from more than one source: although some portion is directly attributable to the illness, other contributing sources are the manner in which the individual patient responds to his or her illness, and the manner in which the system of care and society respond to the circumstances of the patient. These ideas are central in the writings of several British investigators, including Wing and Morris (1981) and Shepherd (1984), who discuss three essential varieties of disability.

PRIMARY DISABILITY

The primary disabilities are those that are associated with illness per se and consist of psychiatric impairments or dysfunctions that may otherwise be described as symptoms of illness. Thus, for example, individuals diagnosed with chronic schizophrenia might exhibit such primary disabilities as lethargy, odd and unacceptable behavior, a lack of awareness of their handicaps, and disturbances in social relationships. It is typically the appearance of these symptoms of illness that leads to diagnosis, and, for many individuals, although not for all, to treatment in the system of care.

Many patient-authors discuss their primary disabilities openly, as shown in this recent posting on the Internet: "I know perfectly well which topics of my thinking are considered delusional by others, and I try not to talk about them in front of people who don't understand that these things are part of 'my reality'" (Naug347@ra.mssstate.edu). Leete (1987), program director for education, advocacy and support at Consumer-Centered Services of Colorado in Denver, describes her hallucinations, suspiciousness, and disorganization in vivid language:

> Sometimes I pace endlessly to relieve the anxiety. I may become frozen in a certain position just because it feels right...[I] curl up, rock back and forth, pace, or become rigid, at times knowing how bizarre this appears.

And McKay (1986), who lives in a shelter for homeless women in Washington, D.C., writes:

> I have been a homeless woman for five years. Sometimes I am sharply aware of my surroundings; sometimes I am like a plastic doll, my staring eyes open but unseeing, or I am like a zombie, moving but unfeeling.

In fact, the importance of accepting one's primary disabilities — one's acknowledgment of illness per se — emerges as a common theme in much of the patient-authored literature. Leete (1987) articulates this idea precisely with the words, "It was not until I had come to accept my illness that I could seriously devise ways of overcoming it."

In this connection some, though certainly not all, patient-authors — perhaps because they are willing and able to acknowledge the their primary disabilities — do not summarily dismiss the need for pharmacotherapies. The literature frequently acknowledges that medications, appropriately prescribed and reviewed, are essential to progress. Leete (1987) writes:

> Despite the embarrassment of troublesome side effects, I now use medication as an adjunct to my other coping mechanisms. However, for many years before I came to realize the role medication could play in the management of my illness, I was caught in a vicious circle. When I was off the medication I couldn't remember how much better I had felt on it, and when I was taking the medication I felt so good that I was convinced I did not need it. Fortunately, through many years of trial and

error, I have now learned what medication works best for me and when to take it to minimize side effects.

Similarly, Harris (1988), notes:

I now must take daily medication. I didn't realize until the last time I went off of it how important the medicine is. Without it, I can't function. It's the difference between being insane and sane.

ADVERSE PERSONAL REACTIONS

In addition to the illness itself, Wing and Morris (1981) and Shepherd (1984) have written about certain adverse personal reactions to illness: secondary disabilities that build upon the primary ones. These secondary disabilities stem not from the illness per se, but rather from the *experience* of illness. Shepherd aptly notes that "a major psychiatric episode is a frightening and disturbing experience and its effects may persist long after the primary symptoms have disappeared." Thus, adverse personal reactions represent an individual patient's idiosyncratic response to his or her own illness.

Many patient-authors agree that adverse personal reactions are of critical importance in the lives of mentally ill persons, a notion that is clearly expressed in an anonymous article appearing in the *American Journal of Psychiatry*:" Even if medication can free the schizophrenic patient from some of his torment, the scars of emotional confusion remain, felt perhaps more deeply by a greater sensitivity and vulnerability" (Recovering Patient, 1986).

Robinson (1983) also offers a very personal account of secondary disabilities:

I was pretty terrified at how far I [had] deteriorated into psychosis...The world of a psychotic is definitely not a pretty one. I remember well the feverish, sleepless nights I spent getting carried away to some magical realm by my own thoughts. My thinking process seemed to me a miracle that could conquer anyone else's. Yet those same thinking processes could overwhelm me into crying oceans of tears over some nostalgic trivia; worse, I could be seized by episodic spasms of sheer unknowable terrors.

Not surprisingly, secondary reactions of despair and sadness are frequently encountered in the literature, as in this poem by Richard B., a patient at Patton State Hospital in California (Wolloch, 1988):

Once upon a time I saw a pterodactyl eating spaghetti.
Above his head the moon cast a shadow on Infinity.
On the earth below a young girl walked barefoot on the damp
grass.

She went to a cave where the ruler of the world lived.
She mustered up enough courage to talk to him.
"Why can't I be happy?" she said to him.
"If I let you be happy, then everyone will want to be happy,"
he said.

Profound frustration and attendant anger are also common themes:

I sound angry — I guess I am — at the illness for invading my
life and making me feel so unsure of myself...at the medical
researchers who now only want to pick and probe into brains
or wherever so they can program measurements into their
computers while ignoring me, the person...at all the literature
which shrouds schizophrenia in negativity, making any
experience connected with it crazy and unacceptable...at the
pharmaceutical industry for being satisfied that their pills keep
me "functional" when all the while I feel drugged and unreal to
myself. And I'm angry at me for believing and trusting too
much in all this information and becoming nothing more than a
patient, a victim of some intangible illness. It's no wonder to
me anymore why I feel I've lost my self, why my existence
seems a waning reflection (McGrath, 1984).

Reactions of fear are also often discussed.

My illness is a journey of fear, often paralyzing, mostly
painful. If only someone could put a bandaid on the
wound...but where? Sometimes I feel I can't stand it any
longer (McGrath, 1984).

Feelings of extreme isolation are frequently addressed in the literature as well. A
patient writing anonymously in the New York Times (Anonymous, 1986) asks,
"Can I ever forget that I am schizophrenic? I am isolated and I am alone. I am
never real. I play-act my life, touching and feeling only shadows." And Beeman
(1984) writes:

> So you end up alone. I think the depression is caused by your isolation, and by the emotional biochemical changes that mental illness causes. It's something you have to experience...It's a painful, yearning kind of thing. It's torture. You yearn to be part of society, but you're locked into your own private prison and you can't get out. It's a terrible thing.

Both Wing and Morris (1981) and Shepherd (1984) have noted that the adverse personal reactions may present as much of a problem for successful engagement and treatment as do the primary symptoms of the illness itself. What is more, since they may endure long after the primary symptoms have abated, they must be fully addressed during treatment.

SOCIAL DISABLEMENTS

Finally, Wing and Morris (1981) and Shepherd (1984) have discussed certain societal events that impose additional disabilities on those who are mentally ill — so-called "social disablements" that are external to the patient. These disabilities come neither from the illness per se nor from personal responses to illness but rather from societal reactions to mental illness.

Leete (1987) provides a particularly succinct and moving description of such tertiary disabilities:

> Sadly, in addition to handicaps imposed by our illnesses, the mentally disabled must constantly deal with barriers erected by society as well. Of these, there is none more devastating, discrediting and disabling to an individual recovering from mental illness than stigma. We are denied jobs, unwanted in our communities. We are seen as unattractive, lazy, stupid, unpredictable, and dangerous.

Some social disablements are quite obvious — for example, inadequate housing markets, stigma, poverty, unemployment, and the general absence of a niche in society. Yet, serious as these are, we are at least able to name them and so, potentially, to consider means for eradicating them. It is, however, the more subtle social disablements — the ones for which we have no names — that most worry many patients as well as many service providers who are involved in mental health program planning.

For example, bureaucratic decisions in federal and state agencies to separate mental health, drug abuse, and alcoholism services may promote unrecognized social disablements (Bachrach, 1987). Because patients often have multiple problems, they may require services offered in all three classes of agencies; and categorical separation of services, far from encouraging comprehensiveness and continuity of care, leads to severe service fragmentation. It may at times even provide extraordinary gatekeeping powers to agencies serving mentally ill persons by legitimizing the exclusion of certain kinds of patients.

The negative consequences of categorical service separation are addressed in a statement by Green (1996):

> My name is Virginia and I am an alcoholic. My name is Virginia and I am a drug addict. My name is Virginia and I am manic-depressive. If it were possible to divide Virginia into three, each illness could be treated according to the traditional yet differing approaches and philosophies of the substance abuse and mental health fields. But alas, or hooray, Virginia is one person. My name is Virginia and I am an alcoholic, drug-addicted person with a major mental illness. For me these disorders are inextricably interconnected. Until I was able to overcome my own denial regarding my substance abuse, I was not able to seek the help I needed. When I had overcome my denial, the help I needed was difficult to find.

In fact, the patient-authored literature is particularly strong in its descriptions of social disablements. Joseph Rogers (1986), chairperson of the National Mental Health Consumers' Association, captures the general sense of that literature in testimony presented before a United States Senate subcommittee:

Over the years, I have found that there is very little understanding in the community of the problem of mental illness, and a lot of fear. There's a great deal of stigma, a negative attitude on the part of the public and, unfortunately, in many communities on the part of public officials. There's a feeling that we must sweep this illness under the rug; we must lock the people away; we must not deal with it.

Unfortunately, stigma may be attached to the very act of taking medications. Collins (1993), a practicing attorney who suffers from bipolar disorder, writes:

> Even though certain brave members of the arts and entertainment industry have come forward to share their experiences with psychiatric medications, the shame in mainstream America prevails...This perverse philosophy is

reinforced by social agencies caring for the less fortunate; in my city, most halfway houses willingly accept recovering alcoholics and addicts, but not those taking psychiatric medications...Many people who take medications live in fear of discovery. Self-disclosure is unthinkable ("I'll lose my job"). So a significant part of their lives remains hidden. That can lead to loneliness, the kind of isolation that was almost deadly for me. My recovery came only with my willingness to open up to others.

RELATIONSHIPS AMONG DISABILITIES

In many of the examples cited here it is difficult to sort out primary, secondary, and tertiary disabilities. Indeed, the patient-authored literature makes a major contribution to the field of program planning through its eloquent reinforcement of a critical point: that sources of disability are separable only in theory and that they are inextricably interwoven in patients' daily lives. The result of this complexity is a milieu filled with pain and despair. The previously cited anonymous author in the *American Journal of Psychiatry* writes:

During times when I am able to recognize...[a] need for closeness, yet remain afraid of it, pushing people away while perceiving them as rejecting me, I struggle with incredible pain. It seems that a great chasm spans between myself and that which I want so much and which I try so hard to get. Even as I write these words I am overcome by what seems the impossibility of closing the gap; I must struggle every day not to lose sight of the fact that I am learning and although I feel stagnant at times and overrun by fears both from within and without, it is indeed possible that one day I will achieve that which I seek (Recovering Patient, 1986)

The same writer is moved to question the unqualified value of treatment:

With the struggles back and forth it almost seems questionable at times whether all this is really worth it. There are days when I wonder if it might not be more humane to leave the schizophrenic patient to his own world of unreality, not to make him go through the pain it takes to become a part of humanity.

DISABILITY AND DIFFICULT PATIENTHOOD

Not only do patient-authors document the inextricable link among the various sources of disability, they go far beyond this to establish that there is also an inescapable relationship between this conceptual field and that of difficult patienthood. Patient-authors thus encourage professionals to ask a basic, but perhaps uncomfortable, question: Are patients burdensome to clinicians and to service systems — i.e., are they difficult patients — because of their illnesses: their primary disabilities? Or might other circumstances account for their lack of cooperation or compliance?

The answer is, of course, a complex one. Certainly, some portion of difficult patienthood resides in illness-related primary symptoms. Yet it seems likely that other major precipitants of patients' apparent intractability are related to the fact that professionals often expect mentally ill people to behave in ways that complicate their clinical courses and exacerbate their disabilities. Clinicians' expectations and service system deficits often conspire to increase patients' secondary and tertiary disabilities and to cause immeasurable pain to them, a point once again underscored simply and forcefully by Leete (1987): "I have come to believe that mental health clients are not treatment-resistant, as is so often stated, but instead only system-resistant."

Thus, it is not enough to offer patients pharmacotherapies that might reduce their symptoms: that respond exclusively to their primary disabilities. Those disabilities most assuredly must be treated, but they are only part of the picture.

Similarly, it is not enough to provide patients with therapies and rehabilitative interventions that might reverse their adverse personal reactions: that might help them respond more appropriately to their illnesses. These kinds of interventions are certainly important, too; but, once again, they are only part of a larger picture.

The patient-authored literature leaves little doubt, in sum, that mental health service systems wishing to respond to the needs of mentally ill individuals must also be sensitive to the societal dimensions of illness. It strongly and definitely supports the notion that service systems must try, as best they can, to mitigate such social disablements as service fragmentation, urban gentrification, limited housing markets, stigma, inadequate health and welfare resources, and even more subtle circumstances that we have not named that profoundly affect what we offer to people who are mentally ill.

INDIVIDUALIZED TREATMENT PLANNING

A third conceptual area influencing mental health program planning today is ou growing understanding of the need for individualized treatments. The fact tha those patients who need the most comprehensive and sophisticated care are ofter given the least individualized treatments has become a source of great concern tc many planners, and it is probably accurate to predict that the future success o mental health programming will depend upon our ability to implement the concepts associated with individualized treatment (Bachrach, 1989).

Once again, statements in the patient-authored literature support this notion often with great poignancy. Willis writes of her stay in a psychiatric hospital "My experience in the hospital was pretty typical: woke up, took medication went to lunch, took medicine, came back to the ward, ate dinner, and took medicine" (California Department of Mental Health, 1989).

However, the lack of individual attention to people's needs is not limited tc hospital settings; it is found in community-based agencies as well. McKay's (1987) words underscore the fact that it is particularly troublesome in facilitie. that serve homeless mentally ill individuals:

> In my view, the big mistake people make in trying to help the homeless is that they expect, or hope, that one single solution will solve the problems of all of us. Generally we, the homeless, are viewed as strands on the same gray mop...My view from the park bench, from the narrow cot in crowded shelters, from the shuffling lines at feeding stations is that we are not all alike by any means and that, in fact, the solution for one of us can spell disaster for another.

SOME NEGLECTED POINTS IN PROGRAM PLANNING

The foregoing observations reveal that, generally speaking, there is considerable concordance between the expressed service needs of patient-authors and the notions that, at least in theory, increasingly inform professional planning efforts This should be gratifying to program planners who have apparently not, from the point of view of patient-authors, gone off into orbits that are removed from thei expressed concerns.

That is the good news. At the same time, however, the patient-authored literature reveals a number of relevant notions and ideas that are at best rarely given credence by professional program planners. Among these are the importance of hope to patients, their need for validation and encouragement, and their wish to be more fully involved in program planning efforts.

The importance of hope is often expressed in poetry, as in these words by a patient at the Rhode Island Institute of Mental Health (1984) who signs her name as Hilda:

> I've got room for friends
> I've got room for sunshine
> I've got room for laughter
> I've got room for fortune
> I've got room for tomorrow

Maria, a patient at the Clarke Institute of Psychiatry in Toronto (1991), also speaks of the importance of hope in a short poem:

> Springtime is here once again,
> about violets I'll remember,
> they are on their way to being.
> I wish they'd last until September,
> my birthday I'd celebrate,
> with a bouquet of flowers so blue,
> and my life would start anew.

And the futility of having no hope is poetically documented in narrative form by Leete (1987):

> We are met by profound silence by all when we ask if we will ever be all right. Imagine our feelings of worthlessness as we are continually bounced from hospital to hospital, transferred from doctor to doctor, switched from one medication to another, and thrown into one living situation after another, making any kind of coordinated or consistent treatment impossible and only convincing us further that our situation is hopeless. The only uniform messages we get from others are that we are incapable of functioning successfully, that we cannot be independent, that we will never get well.

Thus, patient-authored writings strongly emphasize that where there is no hope there can be no improvement: that where there is no hope the individual is doomed to desolation. I have in the course of my professional lifetime reviewed many professionally-authored articles on mental health program planning and will attest that relatively few deal with the idea of hope in any way, shape, or form.

This is true also for discussions of the role of professionals in instilling hope. The patient-authored literature is strong in stating that, in order for hope to flourish, patients must be given a chance by their caregivers. They must be engaged through encouragement and support from professionals who validate their ability to change — a sentiment simply but very forcefully expressed by Peterson (1978), a member of the Fountain House program in New York City: "For me, rehabilitation is not having something done to me."

Still another theme related to hope that is prominent in the patient-authored literature, but once again largely ignored in the professional literature, is the notion that hope is often an outgrowth of a special relationship between patient and therapist. Leighton (1988), director of the Family and Individual Reliance Project for the Mental Health Association of Texas, writes of a particular psychologist:

> She was more human than any of the other doctors I had seen and treated me more humanely. There was a rapport and an equality between us... With the other doctors I had seen, I felt inferior in their presence. Of course, my ego was badly damaged by the illness. But their superior attitudes hurt me even more. This psychologist treated me like one human being helping another. For the first time, strength in me was recognized and fostered. Early in her treatment of me, she let me know I had responsibility over my own illness and wellness. She insisted that I try, something never suggested previously. Her expectations of me and the hard work she demanded on my part are the major reasons I recovered.

Time and time again the patient-authored literature reinforces the reciprocity between establishing a special and productive therapeutic relationship, the emergence of a feeling of acceptance, the birth of hope, and the beginnings of improved functioning. Lovejoy (1984) explains that, when these came together for her, she was able to change her life "through the help of others rather than being a passive victim, and to replace self-pity and helplessness with courage and honesty."

The lesson here for professionals is evident. Since patients' needs and characteristics differ widely, they may possibly have a better prognosis in some other program, in some other place, or with some other clinician. Professional planners must be prepared to acknowledge this circumstance and grant flexibility in program development (Bachrach 1989).

Patient-authors also stress in their writings — and, once again, this emphasis is largely absent from the professional literature, although that has begun to change in recent years — a strong desire to be more fully involved in their own program planning. The failure to consult patients in matters that affect their own welfare is widely perceived among patient-authors as demoralizing and dehumanizing. A patient at the Rhode Island Institute of Mental Health (1984) who signs his name as Gavin describes the hopelessness that results from his inability to control the direction of his life:

> My whole life has been
> Wrapped up in the way
> Doctors, nurses, mental attendants
> Make a discussion over
> How to live my life in the hospital
> I've been in institutions so long
> I can't make a decision
> On my own

For some patient-authors the need for personal involvement in the planning process is expressed as a desire for more mutual help, peer-support, and advocacy (Rogers, 1995). Field (1988) reports on his attendance at a conference organized for former patients: "It's hard to describe how good it feels to be surrounded by hundreds of people who know what you're talking about. It was traveling one thousand miles only to find yourself at home."

ANALYSIS AND CONCLUSIONS

It is important to acknowledge that, although this analysis of patient-authored literature documents some general emphases and perhaps provides tentative direction for program planners, it also contains some serious methodological difficulties. Because the material examined can generate profound personal reactions and can lead to highly subjective conclusions, I have resisted referring to this work as a bona fide content analysis, and I have not presented my findings in a quantitative format. This, of course, makes it difficult to replicate the findings reported here and to verify their validity.

A cautionary word about the generalizability of these findings is also in order. The observations made here should perhaps be understood more as hypothesis-generating statements than as definitive findings, for the literature reviewed for this analysis reflects only the views of those patients or former patients who write, and there is obviously a possibility that they do not represent the majority of mentally ill individuals. On the other hand, these writings most assuredly *do* reflect the thinking of *some* current and former patients; and if we are attempting to listen to what patients have to say, we might as well start with those who, by virtue of their writing, have indicated a willingness and penchant for sharing their thoughts.

Attending to the patient-authored literature, which is obviously a just and humane exercise, is also a sensible thing for professionals to do, for they stand to learn much from the experience. For example, McKay (1986) writes of her stay in a psychiatric ward:

> Drugs every few hours. Forced recreation. Scolding if you lie down too much. Nothing to do but smoke. Boredom. Everyone half-stupefied under medication. The smell of hospital everywhere.

By contrast, life on the streets, though hardly desirable, may offer some meager compensations by comparison:

> There is something to *do* outside [the hospital]. Something to look at. The homeless can go to their favorite corner to beg...Once or twice, if they're lucky begging, they can go for a cup of coffee. They can hope that the next day will be different. They can make plans for themselves...Inside an institution, there is nothing to do for yourself, for your future (McKay, 1986).

Statements like these suggest that homelessness for mentally ill persons more often reflects service system deficits than it does an individual's abstract "choice" to live on the streets. Indeed, an anonymous report by a patient living in Oklahoma addresses the matter of choice directly:

> Someone who has been on the streets and is homeless and jobless and who has a disability, who doesn't have a car or food or a friend, and doesn't know what to do to change their situation, is in pain. Most people would probably agree that if given a choice they would trade that level of emotional pain

for some good old-fashioned physical hurt anytime. But there
is no choice. If you talk to someone who has been there, they
will tell you they were alone and afraid. So afraid that help
doesn't look like help, but like more torture. (Anonymous,
1988)

Professionals who follow the patient-authored literature will also find that the
mental health service system may be different things at different times to
different patients; or even to the same patient at different times — a fact that
service planners frequently overlook. Leighton (1988) writes:

I'm one of the fortunate ones. I learned the hard way that what happens in the
mental health system is not always good for your mental health. But sometimes it
is. And for me, that's made all the difference.

Those in the professional community who are inclined — and often with good
reason — to view the service system as a massive monolith impervious to change
may take heart from these words and be motivated to assume greater flexibility
in their program planning as they respond to this variability.

Perhaps most importantly, however, the patient-authored literature can provide
the professional planner with a heightened sense of the profoundness of patients'
secondary disabilities — the vastness of their shattered hopes and terrible
frustrations. Armed with this knowledge, mental health professionals may wish
to call into question the very language that they employ. For example, Leighton
(1988) writes:

Being called "chronic," as I was, was killing...It made me feel
so helpless and hopeless. It made me want to give up. That's
why as a mental health consumer advocate, I try to help
change the terminology from "chronic" to "long-term."

Many professionals (I among them) see some positive value in using the word
chronic and in not substituting other terminology which will probably turn out to
be just as stigmatizing. They fear, moreover, that playing fast and loose with
language might even have negative consequences by costing patients some of
their entitlements and benefits (Bachrach, 1988). Nonetheless, Leighton's words
carry an undeniable emotional force that may move professionals to understand
that their "neutral" academic approach is really very charged for patients. From
such understanding comes the possibility of change.

Thus, the substantive value of patient-authored literature is considerable, for it is replete with perspectives that are relevant to mental health program planning that may be advantageously exploited by the professional community. Patient-authored writings generate a heightened awareness of the complexities surrounding relevant and sensitive service delivery and underscore the fact that services for mentally ill persons must consist of much more than prefabricated program elements selected from a menu of offerings. They must be constructed with full appreciation of the needs and hopes of the individuals who are to be served.

REFERENCES

Allen, P. (1974) "A consumer's view of California's mental health care system". *Psychiatric Quarterly*, 48, 1–13.

Anonymous (1986) "I feel I am trapped inside my head, banging against its walls, trying desperately to escape". *New York Times*, March 18.

Anonymous (1988, Summer) "Someone who has been there". *Newsletter of New Beginnings*, Elgin, Oklahoma, unpaginated.

Bachrach, L.L. (1987) "The chronic mental patient with substance abuse problems". In *New Directions for Mental Health Services no. 35: Leona Bachrach Speaks* (pp. 29–41) San Francisco, CA: Jossey-Bass.

Bachrach, L.L. (1988) "Defining chronic mental illness: a concept paper". *Hospital and Community Psychiatry*, 398, 383–388.

Bachrach, L.L. (1989) "The legacy of model programs". *Hospital and Community Psychiatry*, 40, 234–235.

Bachrach, L.L., Talbott, J.A., and Meyerson, A.T. (1987) "The chronic psychiatric patient as a 'difficult' patient: a conceptual analysis". In, *"New Directions for Mental Health Services", no. 33: Barriers to Treating the Chronic Mentally Ill* (pp. 35–50) (ed. Meyerson A.T.) Jossey-Bass, San Francisco, CA.

Beeman, R. (1984 October 2) "You're sort of trapped in this inner world in seeds of crisis". *Special Report of the Mesa-Tempe-Chandler (Arizona) Tribune*, September 28-October 2, 1988, p. 4.

Blaska, B: (1994) "How to treat inpatients". Letter to *Hospital and Community Psychiatry* , 45, 1239–1240.

Brundage, B.E. (1983) "First Person Account: What I Wanted to Know but was Afraid to Ask", *Schizophrenia Bulletin,* 8, 583–585.

California Department of Mental Health (1989) *People Say I'm Crazy,* Sacramento CA: Department of Mental Health.

Chrzanowski, G. (1980) "Problem patients or troublemakers? Dynamic and therapeutic considerations", *American Journal of Psychotherapy,* 34, 26–38

Clarke Institute of Psychiatry (1991) *Windows and Mirrors: Poetry and Stories Created by Patients,* Toronto: Clarke Institute of Psychiatry.

Collier, T.J. (1993) "The Stigma of Mental Illness", *Newsweek,* 26 April.

Field, T. (1988, September/October) *Salt Lake City Conference Peak Experience for Consumers,* Spotlight (Newsletter published by Washington Advocates for the Mentally Ill, Seattle), no. 11, unpaginated.

Green, V.L. (1996)   "The Resurrection and the Life", *American Journal of Orthopsychiatry,*   66, 12–16.

Harris, M. & Bergman, H.C. (1986-87) "The narcissistically vulnerable system: a case study of the public mental hospital", *Psychiatry Quarterly,* 58, 202–212.

Harris, N. (1988) "A personal history from a case management program client", *Psychosocial Rehabilitation Journal,* 11, 58–62.

Jeffry, R. (1979) "Normal rubbish: deviant patients in casualty departments", *Sociology of Health and Illness,* 1, 90–107.

Leete, E. (1987, October) "Overcoming mental illness: a survivor's perspective",   Paper presented at the Institute of Hospital and Community Psychiatry, Boston.

Leighton D.C. (1988) "Being mentally ill in America: one female's experience",   In, *Treating Chronically Mentally Ill Women* (L.L. & Nadelson C.C. eds.) pp. 63-73. American Psychiatric Press , Washington, D.C.,.

Lovejoy, M. (1984)   "Recovery from schizophrenia: a personal odyssey", *Hospital and Community Psychiatry,* 1984, 809–812.

McGrath, M.E. (1984) "First person account: Where did I go"? *Schizophrenia Bulletin,* 638-640.

McKay, P. (1986, February 16) "My home is a lonely bed in a dreary D.C. shelter", Washington Post, pp. C1, C3.

McKay, P. (1987, December 29) "We bag ladies aren't all alike", *Washington Post*, pp. C1, C2.

Naug347@ra.msstate.edu. (1996) "Posting to Internet schizophrenia discussion", Group, 31 January

Neill J.R. (1979) "The difficult patient: identification and response", *Journal of Clinical Psychiatry*, 40, 209–212.

Peterson, R. (1978) "What are the needs of chronic mental patients"? In *The Chronic Mental Patient: Problems, Solutions and Recommendations for a Public Policy* (eds. Talbott J.A.) pp. 39–49. American Psychiatric Association, Washington, D.C.

Recovering Patient. (1986) "Can we talk?" The schizophrenic patient in psychotherapy, *American Journal of Psychiatry* 143, 68–70.

Rhode Island Institute of Mental Health. (1984) *Mindscapes*, Cranston, RI: Rhode Island Institute of Mental Health.

Robinson, B.P. (1983, April 3) "When I finally realized I was insane", *Washington Post*, pp. D1, D2.

Rogers, J.A. (1986, November 20) *Testimony Presented at Hearings on Schizophrenia*, United States Senate Subcommittee on Labor, Health and Human Services Education, Washington

Rogers, J.A. (1995) Community organizing: self help and providing mental health Services. *Journal of the California Alliance for the Mentally Ill*, 6, 41–43.

Ruocchio, P.J. (1987) "Perils of social development for the schizophrenic patient", *Hospital and Community Psychiatry*, 38, 1223–1224.

Sharp, M.L. (1988, April 14) "Life without stelazine" Paper presented at San Francisco General Hospital Psychiatric Grand Rounds, San Francisco.

Shepherd, G. (1984) *Institutional Care and Rehabilitation*. London: Longman.

Weinberg, J. (1978) "The chronic patient: the stranger in our midst", *Hospital and Community Psychiatry*, 29, 25–28.

Wing, J.K., & Morris, B. (1981) "Clinical basis of rehabilitation". In *Handbook of Psychiatric Rehabilitation Practice* (eds. Wing J.K. & Morris B.), Oxford University Press, England.

Wolloch, C. (Ed.)(1988) *The Shrill Cry of the Muse: Poems from Patton State Hospital.* Patton CA: Patton State Hospital.

3

WORK AND MENTAL ILLNESS: TOWARD AN INTEGRATION OF TREATMENT AND REHABILITATION

Courtenay M. Harding, John S. Strauss, Hisham Hafez, and Paul B. Lieberman

In 172 AD, Galen pronounced that: "Employment is nature's best physician and is essential to human happiness" (in Strauss, 1968, p. 663). Over the centuries, the view that work is crucial to mental health and to the treatment of mental illness has persisted (Freud, 1930/1953; Kirkbride, in Bond, 1947; Kraepelin, 1902). Despite this basic understanding of human functioning, the integration of work into systems which treat severe mental illness is limited, sporadic, and inadequately addressed.

Divisions between the treatment and rehabilitation systems often stem from widely differing theoretical, training, and administrative orientations which have focused persistently on narrow and often separate concerns (Anthony and Buell, 1973; Strauss et al., 1988). Industrial psychologists have described the interface between the characteristics of the job and those of the workers for specific subgroups of the general population (Dunnette, 1976; Early, 1973; Posner and Randolph, 1979; Thorndike, 1949). Additional focus has been placed on the impact of working relationships, such as co-workers and supervisors, at the work site (Berger, 1964; Rosenthal, 1978; Zaleznick, 1965). Vocational rehabilitation and occupational therapy efforts have targeted the development and study of a wide variety of innovative and traditional programs as a primary concern (Beard et al., 1982; Black, 1976; Fairweather, 1969; Rennie et al., 1950). Additional

Schizophrenia: Breaking Down the Barriers. Edited by S.G. Holliday, R.J. Ancill and G.W. MacEwan. © 1996 John Wiley & Sons Ltd

investigations of psychiatric patients have also been conducted to assess attitudes (Burke and Sellin, 1972; Hartlage, 1967), clarify cognitive processes (Mordock and Feldman, 1969), measure performance (Cheadle et al., 1967; Dilling et al., 1973; Griffiths, 1973), document outcome (Anthony et al., 1978; Cole and Shupe, 1970; Paul, 1984; Strauss and Carpenter, 1974), and evaluate programs (Dellario, 1982; Loeb et al., 1974; Stein and Test, 1980; Walker, 1979). Most of this work based its primary assumptions on the theoretical frameworks provided by either the Rehabilitation Model (Anthony, 1979 a; Rusk and Taylor, 1949) or the Social Learning Model (Bandura and Walters, 1963; Liberman et al, 1986). These models emphasize interventions to improve function, to compensate for impairment, disability, and handicap, or to reshape the surrounding environment. They do not focus on the nature of the disorders leading to impairment or on the continued interaction of illness characteristics with the process of returning to work.

Investigators, operating within illness models, have taken a divergent path (Strauss and Carpenter, 1981). They have focused either on concepts of etiology, evolving course of disorder, underlying vulnerability, limits of stimulation, or the resolution of conflicts. Further, studies have targeted work as related to prognosis in severe psychiatric disorders (Huffine and Clausen, 1979; Strauss and Carpenter, 1977; Strauss and Chen, 1977), work in connection with the social outcome of mental illness (Bleuler, 1972/1978; Chittick et al., 1961; Ciompi and Müller, 1976; Clausen, 1975; Tsuang et al., 1979), and work in regard to specific theoretical positions which utilize single case studies as illustrations (Freud, 1930/1953; Hendrick, 1943; Menninger, 1942; White, 1959). Vocational rehabilitation of the psychiatrically disabled person has not been viewed as part of the treatment process, but as something for someone else to do *after* treatment (Anthony and Margules, 1974). However, there has been very little systematic research up to now which has focused on the evolving course of recovery from a severe psychiatric illness, and, in fact, the ingredients which shape that course are far from delineated (Strauss, 1982). The implicit assumption that work cannot be part of treatment remains unwarranted.

These differences in perception and strategies as well as lack of basic knowledge have left both the medical and rehabilitation fields serving the same population of patients, but proceeding in tandem with little understanding of the possible synergistic and beneficial effects of collaboration or of the methods for establishing such a collaboration.

To clarify the nature of this kind of fragmentation and the impact upon the provision of vocational services for persons with mental illness, this chapter reports a survey of the major vocational rehabilitation components available within a mental health system. The survey focused on one community and the degree to which vocational rehabilitation was integrated into its network of care for psychiatric patients. The interviews identified major issues and characteristics of each part of the system which helped or hindered the process of treatment and its vocational rehabilitation components.

METHODS

For this survey, information was obtained from diverse sources in the community. Informants included clinicians, counselors, clients, and families. Observations were made of programs and work sites. Additional outside resources were utilized to widen the perspective.

PROGRAMS

The major rehabilitation service providers within one geographic area (New Haven, CT) were selected. Greater New Haven, with its adjacent twelve towns, comprised a catchment area of 420,021 people (Tischler et al, 1972, 1975). The purpose of these rehabilitation programs was to facilitate patients' entry or re-entry into a work situation following an episode of severe mental illness. Descriptions of vocational rehabilitation in the literature and from colleagues in various parts of the United States revealed that the programs under study represented the more progressive end of the spectrum. They were located in an above-average mental health and rehabilitation system which had a wide range of components in place. The programs included the following types shown in Table 1.

SURVEY INFORMANTS

1.   Program Administrators and Staff Members
This group included psychologists, social workers, rehabilitation counselors, program directors, and psychiatrists.

2.   Clients
Twenty-eight patients, subjects of the Yale Longitudinal Work Study, also participated (Strauss et al., 1985). They were between 18 and 55, had had a recent inpatient stay for functional psychiatric disorder, no evidence of severe substance abuse/organic brain damage, and had been employed at least part of the year prior to admission. As workers, they didn't represent the entire spectrum of patients with psychiatric illness, but did follow a wide variety of trajectories in their post-episode courses, ranging from those with total unemployment for 2 years to those who returned to work while still hospitalized at night.

TABLE 1. Major Rehabilitation Service Providers

Umbrella Agency	Program	Components of Program	Goals of Program
Mental Health Center	Patient-employee work program	Paid positions in selected jobs from food service, plant operation, and mail room.	To be evaluated and trained in 18 months as mandated by state DMH
Veterans administration hospital	Veterans resource program	In-hospital work program	To achieve vocational/social rehabilitation and housing in 13 weeks.
Private 66-bed psychiatric facility	Community work adjustment program	Volunteer placements under supervision	To experience work settings under supervision, moving out in 3 months to unsupervised community placement
Private nonprofit rehabilitation facility	Work adjustment program	Each client provided with individual work plan; supervision in a warehouse completing outside work contracts	To promote an understanding of responsibilities of competitive employment; to develop appropriate personal characteristics, work behaviours, and concrete skills; reviewed every 3 months
	Occupational skills training program	Supervised in a clerical office and entry-level computer programming	To develop marketable and competing work skills and placement; re-evaluated once a month
	Projects with industry	Pre-screening evaluation, job seeking, placement, follow-up, training, post-employment support	To provide area employers with qualified personnel: to offer persons with disabilities a chance for personal and financial rewards of employment
District office of state agency providing vocational rehabilitation	Vocational rehabilitation	Medical and psychological evaluation; vocational counseling and guidance; physical and mental restorative services; vocational training; job placement (selective placement to serve the severely disabled).	To prepare for, obtain, and maintain employment

3. Families
Many relatives of the Yale Work Study subjects, as well as other families in the community whose relatives were in- or out-patients receiving mental health and or rehabilitation services, were also interviewed.

4. Employers
Those who were hiring patients in a wide variety of capacities as well as those employers who were skeptical of doing so shared their opinions as well.

5. Outside Resources
Further information was contributed by families of psychiatric patients through their questions, suggestions, and discussions at state and national conferences of the Alliance for the Mentally Ill (National Alliance for the Mentally Ill, 1984) as well as by William Anthony and his co-workers at Boston University Center for Rehabilitation Research and Training in Mental Health.

PROCEDURE

In the interviews of all service provider informants, a series of questions was asked about the nature and scope of programs and the type of client served. A special focus was placed on which ingredients seemed to promote or discourage optimal vocational program practice (finding the right job for the right person at the right time in the course of recovery from severe psychiatric disorder). See Table 2 for survey categories.

The subjects in the Yale Work Study provided information for this report as part of their participation in a systemic research protocol which utilized a comprehensive semi-structured instrument battery described at length elsewhere (Breier and Strauss, 1983, 1984; Harding and Strauss, 1985; Strauss et al., 1985). An initial series of baseline evaluations was completed during inpatient admission with follow-up interviews every two months for a year and a final interview two years after discharge. Data were collected about the struggles of psychiatrically impaired adults who were trying to adapt once again to community life.

To provide still other perspectives, discussions were held with family members of patients with severe mental disorders. The Boston University Research and Training Center leadership and staff provided another resource of information and opinions. These interviews centered around conceptual and programmatic overviews of the field (e.g. Anthony, 1979a).

TABLE 2. Categories of Inquiry

Programs

1. Characteristics of umbrella agency

a.   Types of services offered
b.   Capacity
c.   Number of patients served in a year
d.   Targeted population
e.   Types of professional personnel
f.   Stated model of treatment
g.   Operation model of treatment
h.   Funding sources

2. Components of specific programs

a.   Types of services offered
b.   Entry criteria
c.   Number of patients served in 1 year
d.   Referral sources
e.   Goals of p program
f.   Stated and operating models of treatment

Clinicians and Counselors

1.   Discipline
2.   Adequacy of original training
3.   Treatment model
4.   Perceived required tasks
5.   Actual performed services
6.   Perceptions of ways in which the current system helps or hinders process of treatment/rehabilitation
7.   Experience with families

Clients

1.   Work and illness histories
2.   current episode descriptions
3.   Work and structure
4.   Work and self-esteem
5.   Work and social supports
6.   Work and treatment
7.   Work and symptoms
8.   Work and degree of involvement
9.   Work and other life contexts
10. Impact of unemployment
11. Experience with rehabilitation service services
12. Experience with mental health system
13. What helps and hinders process of recovery

Families

1.   Concepts of work and mental illness
2.   Concerns about current status
3.   Experience with mental health and rehabilitation service providers
4.   Concerns about loved one's future
5.   What helps and what hinders the process

Employers

1.   Concepts and concern about mental illness
2.   Experience with patients and other employers
3.   Experience with mental health and rehabilitation service providers
4.   Experience with other state agencies' requirements as well as with labor unions
5.   What helps and what hinders process

RESULTS

The results of this survey have been organized by two methods. The first strategy describes important issues, counter-productive practices, and solutions encountered by components of the rehabilitation and treatment systems at their interface. These characteristics were grouped by the type of person or the part of the system in which they were the most distinctive (the programs, the people providing rehabilitation and treatment, the clients, the families, and the employers).

The second method focused on an overview which elicited the major impediments to progress that were common across all components.

MAJOR ISSUES, GENERAL PRACTICE, AND COUNTERPRODUCTIVE ACTIVITIES ENCOUNTERED BY SYSTEM COMPONENTS AT THEIR INTERFACE

1. Agency Programs

Rehabilitation programs provided a series of graded steps to promote job re-entry. These steps included such programs as: resocialization, activities of daily living, work activities, sheltered workshops, inhouse training programs, work adjustment, volunteer placement, apprenticeships, job skills training, evaluation, and placement in probationary and competitive employment. Although most of the major programmatic elements were in place within the community, they were widely scattered and poorly linked. Further, these scattered elements did indeed operate in tandem and not in parallel with the mental health treatment system, adding more validity to the literature reviewed.

The mental health system focused its treatment efforts on improved social functioning and symptom reduction using psychopharmacology and approaches to personal and/or family dynamics. There was tacit recognition that patients had spent varying degrees of time in their lives as "workers" (or might possibly become workers, there also appeared to be a relationship between the kind of work a patient did and exacerbation or diminution of symptoms. However, this knowledge was often ranked as secondary in importance to the clinical picture.

As discharge planning was undertaken, clinicians made only infrequent referrals to a vocational rehabilitation program. Those patients who were referred then entered into a different system. They were now viewed as disabled workers rather than disabled persons. This new system operated under a different model. Its stated goals were to assess the worker for the degree of impairment, disability, or handicap; evaluate the person with a battery of measures to determine areas of ability, interests, and skilled performance; send the client to rehabilitation training in order to "get ready to begin;" then on to job training and eventually a job. The complexity and rigidity of the programs at the system interface led to the force-fit of clients to the programs rather than to the individualization of treatment for specific clients (a goal highly touted and rarely accomplished). There was a repeated situation of an overabundance of clients and insufficiently funded programs. This situation placed the focus on only the "guaranteed" successes in vocational placement and job maintenance. Further cuts in training monies set the stage for pushing some clients ahead too quickly or leaving whole classes of people out of programs entirely. The waiting lists demoralized clients, families, and staff. When placement in a program finally occurred, the client was often trained in outmoded job skills on old equipment or for soon-to-be obsolete jobs.

2.   Clinicians and Counselors

Major problems were apparent in linkages between clinical and rehabilitative personnel. There appeared to be little interaction between psychiatrist/psychologist clinicians and rehabilitation counselors. If any interaction occurred, it was often unidirectional and paternalistic in the form of a medical or psychological report to the counselor, and often in terms unsuitable for translation into the concrete work world. The clinicians considered themselves as providing the "treatment." Often the counselor was perceived to be performing an ancillary role. Many clinicians stated that they were not educated on how to make a functional assessment of patient competencies, or were unaware of most existing rehabilitation programs. Therefore, they were unable to communicate effectively with rehabilitation counselors. Further linkage-type pursuits were generally not reimbursed. Thus, busy clinicians resented performing more tasks on their own time.

For rehabilitation workers, high levels of frustration, a sense of isolation from clinical staff, and a pervasive feeling of second-class status were consistently reported, especially among those counselors working within larger medically-oriented treatment centers (Lamb and Mackota, 1975). Rehabilitation personnel frequently reported uneasiness engendered by the lack of formal training in tasks related specifically to the rehabilitation of the psychiatrically disabled person. Skills garnered from previous training in other fields such as physical disability were only of moderate use, so that length of experience with psychiatric clients and a certain dogged persistence appeared to be the critical variables for success. Other salient issues for clinicians and counselors included the counselors' distinct preference for specific compositions of client caseloads (e.g. all alcoholics). The style of interaction with clients was often confrontational and involved free-wheeling decision making, even in the absence of systematic evidence or feedback regarding the efficacy of such decisions or style of interaction.

3. Clients

Clients served by the programs ranged in age from 15 to 65. In addition to having the primary diagnoses of severe, symptomatic mental illness, many clients were also judged to be multiply handicapped by personality disorders, mental retardation, poverty, and the lack of social skills, previous work experience, or education.

This heterogeneity of backgrounds brought together, into the same system, clients who ranged from illiterates to college graduates and from persons with no work history to those with extensive experiences. Programs often grouped together a wide spectrum of clients who displayed heterogeneity of illness characteristics such as different diagnoses, single or multiple diagnoses for the same person, one illness episode vs. multiple episodes, and various degrees of severity. Rather than taking the differences into account when deciding where to place, what to provide, and how quickly to move people around the system, many groups of clients were treated the same in a generic fashion and most were started slowly at point A.

To add to the complexity, clients' needs for specific kinds of person - illness-environment interactions shifted over time as they returned to work during recovery from an episode (Strauss et al., 1985). Thus, for one person, multiple concurrent jobs were found to have an organizing effect, where for another person such a situation was disorganizing. Some subjects returned to work quite early in their recovery period, using work as a buffer while other subjects waited through a long moratorium or "woodshedding" period of convalescence prior to returning to work (The woodshedding concept, taken from the ways jazz musicians practice new music "out of the woodshed," was suggested by P. Lieberman and applied to patients by Joshua Sparrow, M.D., in his unpublished thesis entitled Woodshedding: A Phase in Recovery from Psychosis; Yale University Medical School, New Haven, Connecticut, 1985). Some people initially flourished with a highly structured job which reduced symptoms. Later, the same job became often noxious and exacerbated symptoms when the client's need for structure lessened.

Among other ingredients important in selecting a job at a particular time in the person's course were issues of self-esteem, the meaning of work, better income, and the need for more or less social contacts (Breier and Strauss, 1984). The delicate interplay between all of these forces appeared to promote or obstruct return to health and functioning. It was often difficult for program staff to note and monitor differences in client needs as well as changes in functioning over time which required alteration of employment conditions. Other critical issues add to the picture at the interface of the client with the system.

Clients often displayed unrealistic goals by thinking that they could go out and work an 8-hour day when they had not worked for 10 years. Counselors, on the other hand, often underestimated the clients' potential or the time needed to get geared up to work. Work habits such as arriving to work on time, being neat, and getting along with others were often ignored in preference to job skill training. However, loss of job was attributed more often to lack of these aforementioned social skills. Symptom exacerbation often was seen as a failure of the client, the counselor, and/or the program, but not as part of an episodic illness process.

4.   Families

The families interviewed by the project investigators, as well as those described by the clinicians and counselors, revealed another important part of the vocational rehabilitation process. Aging parents were worried about the seemingly permanent dependence of their offspring and concerned about who would take care of their son or daughter when the parents themselves died. Such families saw the acquisition of a job as a major sign that their ill child was becoming well and assuming the responsibilities of adulthood.

Although most family members assisted clients in crucial ways, clinicians and counselors often viewed families, in general, as either impediments or peripheral to the treatment and rehabilitation process. Many clinicians and counselors entered into either a covert struggle or open warfare with family members over the patient. On the other hand, some families appeared to sabotage the efforts of clients moving toward greater independence. These families created obstacles such as objecting to their grown child learning to ride a bus, insisting on driving the client to the program, or forbidding him or her to travel to a work site. Other issues related to family members had to do with a general lack of understanding about mental illness, particularly negative symptoms, such as apathy and withdrawal. Counselors often assumed that families had this knowledge and covertly or overtly blamed the family either for an etiological role in the patient's illness or in the perpetuation of the pathological process. Many families felt puzzled hurt, angry, guilty, overwhelmed, and isolated. Counselors and clinicians often tried to treat clients as if they were living in a vacuum. As a result, many possible collaborative enterprises were often aborted.

5. The Work Site

Employers appeared to need much the same kind of supports, education, and linkages as those required by families in order to cope with and help people with disabling psychiatric disorders. As with many lay people, employers harbored myths, misinformation, and fears. Mental illness was considered to be an invisible disability (unlike the impairments of a person in a wheelchair) and was difficult to understand. Employer resentment grew over the behaviors displayed by recovering psychiatric patients without obvious handicaps who were trying to re-enter the job market. Social withdrawal was seen as lack of interest and psychomotor retardation seen as laziness, much in the same ways that some untrained families react to the negative symptoms of schizophrenia (Anderson et al., 1980; Vaughn and Leff, 1976). Further, small employers who offered the best chance of flexible supervision were often swamped with federal and state paperwork. Intermittent episodes of illness interrupted job commitment and left employers without a person to do the job. Supervisors were often impersonal or inappropriate. Problems in the economy reduced the number of available jobs, leaving overcredentialed people to fill entry-level openings. Unions feared that the reduced salary and modified job contracts would displace union workers and undermine the union stand on salaries and job descriptions. Sheltered work settings modeled on mental retardation strategies tended not to be as appropriate for people with mental illness. Often there was tacit permission for clients to act in a nonbusinesslike manner, and many clients remained indefinitely in a program that was meant to be a transitional placement.

There are several strategies which appeared to be effective for employers. One of these was employed by a rehabilitation facility, which offered a free consultation about the removal of architectural barriers for the physically handicapped in order to gain entry into the work place and then provided additional educational programs about mental disabilities. Employers' fears that a client would lose control and hurt others, equipment, or self were often alleviated by providing hot lines to responsive counselors and arranging on-site consultation to deal with strange behaviors. Employers' concerns that they would be stuck with a poorly functioning employee were considerably lessened by a contract with the rehabilitation counselor, who agreed to screen, retrain, and fire an unsuccessful employee if necessary. Under those conditions, employers were often willing to try another candidate from the same program.

AN OVERVIEW OF THE TREATMENT–REHABILITATION INTERFACE

The survey has identified four serious impediments to the integration of vocational rehabilitation strategies into the mental health system. The obstacles include: rigidity, isolation, compensatory ad hoc operations, and narrow frames of reference. These themes are repeated at each interface of the system components.

Rigidity

A major inhibitor to progress appeared to be a lack of flexibility found in theoretical models, system design, and treatment modalities, as well as in expectations for clients. This rigidity pervaded the process and inhibited the attainment of the treatment/rehabilitation goals.

Mental health and rehabilitation programs were often heavily structured with copious procedures and rules. Potentially dynamic and creative clinicians and counselors were blocked by voluminous paperwork, inflexible time frames, adherence to the manual, and the need to produce "closed" cases. Both sides of the system shuffled people along its course regardless of individual needs, sometimes holding people for great lengths of time because of evaluation, training, and placement procedures. There were waiting lists and gaps of service. Clients as well as clinicians/counselors often felt devalued, isolated, and burned out.

Isolation

The community which this report has focused had a wide range of services available, but these services were poorly linked in many cases. Costly duplication of programs occurred, and clients who were lost to follow-up or who fitted programs poorly, consumed precious resources, while not receiving the help for which the system was established.

Families, as well as clients, were often shut out of most major decisions affecting the trajectory of treatment. Many were attempting to wend their way through a complicated network without knowing which options were offered by the system components. The wealth of other knowledge and expertise was often not requested by clinicians or counselors, who regarded such information about personal responses to illness characteristics, medications, coping strategies, and life goals as decidedly idiosyncratic, mostly pathological, and/or simply not useful.

Ad Hoc Compensatory Operations

An improvised nonsystem emerged to cope with the rigidity and lack of an overarching understanding of how work affects the course of severe psychiatric disorder. This non-system relied heavily on the ingenuity of counselors or clinicians who subverted the process in order to achieve client-centered goals. Bringing into day-to-day practice every ounce of experience, assorted skills, and personal interconnections across agencies, these workers spent countless hours laboring outside the system to achieve linkages, medical treatment, and rehabilitation for their clients. However, flying-by-the-seat-of-one's-pants often led to an undermining lack of professional identity among the counselors, a one-down position when dealing with their medical counterparts undifferentiated concepts, and an unwitting use of personal values in the interpretation of clients' needs.

Narrow Frames of Reference

Although the members of each component of the system had acquired skills and experience over the years, they still operated as groups of separate disciplines. Many clinicians knew very little about rehabilitation or even how to write an adequate referral for a rehabilitation program. In a narrow application of the medical model, clinicians often failed to appreciate that work or vocational rehabilitation might have an impact on symptom relief or on the course of disorder. On the other hand, counselors were often not educated about clinical issues, other treatment modalities, or even about mental illness itself, and usually focused on decreasing skill deficits. Families and clients suffered as well from lack of a more general framework including education about mental illness and vocational rehabilitation.

DISCUSSION

Analysis of the different components of the overall system which provided mental health and vocational rehabilitation services to the provided mental health and vocational rehabilitation services to the same client population suggested a variety of solutions to the problems of rigidity, isolation, ad hoc compensatory operations, and narrow frames of reference. These solutions can be grouped under four headings: flexibility, collaboration, data-based training, and a unified theoretical framework.

FLEXIBILITY

From all perspectives, observation of clients repeatedly indicates the need for flexibility across the interface of components in the system. Clients often progress slowly, then pick up tempo as their illnesses lift (Harding et al., 1987a, b, c). As people with heterogeneous skills, aptitudes, and severity of illnesses, they need to go up and down through graded services and often in and out of them. Life proceeds, and even with an on-going disorder and unchanged medication, clients acquire experience and undergo changes in attitudes, perceptions, feelings of self-esteem, skills, and supports.

Flexibility includes restructuring the system around these changing client needs and incorporating longitudinal perspectives and strategies to deal with psychiatric illnesses which occur episodically across long periods of a life course. Such an approach represents a substantial shift from crisis intervention and custodial care techniques.

Flexibility in systems becomes difficult when resources are scarce, many governmental regulations, and when there are large numbers of clients to serve. However, current programs proceed only because of unrelenting commitment and hard work on the part of individuals and because of overt, as well as covert, circumvention of the rigid framework.

COLLABORATION

Collaboration within and across agencies and participants in the treatment/rehabilitation system is essential. One solution proposed is an overriding consortium of agency programs which would begin to bridge the gap between them. Two such consortia have been established recently in the community under assessment. One is called the Consortium for Community Support Programs, and is composed of the management levels from sixteen agencies. The other has been established by rehabilitation workers who represent twenty-five agencies and is named the Rehabilitation Consortium of Greater New Haven. Linkages have improved substantially.

Increased collaborations at other levels are important as well. Those clinicians and counselors, who cross-train each other, learn to speak a common language and to work together on behalf of the same client for whom they share responsibility. Working together in partnership with the client (who often has to be taught to undo the passive role frequently fostered by the system), this team can promote individualized and comprehensive treatment plans. These plans are then more congruent with the client's needs and goals.

Collaboration with families is on approach just beginning to be utilized. Family members working as a part of the enterprise on behalf of the client can facilitate the healing process. Furthermore, educating families about what a mental health care delivery system needs to treat their afflicted member empowers families to educate legislative appropriations committees for increased funding (Disher, 1985). Increasingly, families are seen as the truly "interested" parties by legislatures and not as self-serving mental health professional lobbies (Bernheim, 1987). Collaboration between employers and treatment teams who educate each other and provide back-up support also has been shown to be effective in maintaining clients in jobs (Magee et al., 1982).

DATA-BASED TRAINING

The education of the various participants in the system has proceeded from narrow conceptions generated by specific disciplines or from acquired life experiences. Each discipline has produced some evidence for its position about cause, course, and treatment of mental illness, but without follow-up research to document and demonstrate various aspects of program efficacy or lack of it, the feedback loop to shape and test intuitions is nearly absent. Further, there is a startling paucity of longitudinal empirical evidence (Strauss, et al., 1985) about illness characteristics such as natural periodicity, the active role of the patient, the acquisition of self-control mechanisms, the role of work, and many other variables which appear to shape, buffer, and modulate the course of illness over time (Breier and Strauss, 1983; Strauss et al., 1988). Until these data are acquired, we will continue to operate in the semi-darkness.

A UNIFIED THEORETICAL FRAMEWORK

Collaboration, flexibility, and data-based training across components of the system lead naturally to the need of an overarching model for the rehabilitation of the mentally ill. Each caregiver, whether clinician or rehabilitation counselor, focuses on different aspects of the same client. These aspects interact within the client and influence outcome in all spheres such as psychological, social, and occupational functioning. For example, if "disabled workers" become "able workers," their self-esteem often increases, their support systems may widen, and their resources for coping are enhanced. In many cases, these factors have helped patients to tolerate some unresolved stresses and may have reduced the possibility of a relapse. Likewise, if "disabled patients" become more "able persons," then this sense of efficacy may overflow into their role of workers, doubling the benefit. Knitting together the theoretical framework involves both clinical and rehabilitative orientations.

However, inhibitions to such a goal lie in the fact that clinicians and rehabilitation counselors are drawn from many professions (e.g., counseling programs, social work, psychology, nursing, and psychiatry). Each of these disciplines has its own model which specifically shapes a view of patients, treatment, and illness. To add to the confusion, several models may be covertly utilized even within one discipline (Lazare, 1973). Although some investigators view the medical model with its orientation toward pathology as competing with and often counter-productive to the competence goals of rehabilitation efforts (Albee, 1969; Blaney, 1975; Ryan et al., 1982), others have proposed either a wider application of the existing medical model (Adler, 1981) or a more comprehensive rehabilitation model (Anthony, 1979) to solve a problem.

On one hand, Astrachan et al., (1976) proposed to incorporate the medical, rehabilitative, societal-legal, and educative developmental perspectives and tasks under the umbrella of psychiatry as interconnected and sanctioned by society. On the other hand, Anthony (1979 a & b), has pioneered in developing an expanded rehabilitation model for the psychiatrically disabled person. Anthony (1979b) targeted an assessment of functional abilities and environmental demands. Anthony (1982) was influenced by the rehabilitation model for the physically ill, such as those described by Rusk and Taylor (1949). The BU team (Anthony et al., 1984) has stated that psychiatric rehabilitation is "atheoretical and eclectic." Anthony et al. (1984), Grob (1983), Dincin (1981), and others have meant "atheoretical" in terms of the etiology of mental illness. However, in practice, rehabilitation is actually carried out by methods based on specific theories and concepts about mental illness learned in the caregiver's original discipline and heavily modified by the predominant model of the agency in which the service is being rendered.

Whether starting from a medical or a rehabilitation model, it continues to be difficult in practice, as well as theory, to combine notions of disorder and competence in a truly integrated fashion. As if this was not enough of a problem, the agency's philosophy of rehabilitation and health care delivery is determined by local, state, and federal priorities and reimbursement policies. Thus, without a strong comprehensive model, the effect of any individual construct is washed away by stronger currents, leaving a fragmented system of care.

If rehabilitation is to be carried out in an integrated manner, its roles and linkages within the broader conception must be developed (Cohen, 1981).

Consideration of the best ingredients from the knowledge base acquired by each of the various disciplines involved in day-to-day practice point the way to a combined, more complete framework. The development of an integrated model for the entire field of psychiatric rehabilitation must include an understanding of course of illness, prognosis, the role of competence, and biological interaction with the person and his or her environment. The beginnings of such models have been proposed by Strauss and Carpenter in their Interactive Developmental Model (1981), Engel's Biopsychosocial Model (1977 & 1980), and Astrachan et al.'s (1976) Expanded Medical Model. The best known program, that attempts such an integration is the Training in Community Living Program in Madison, Wisconsin, conducted by Stein and Test (1980).

The basic groundwork in the field has been established, but until the next step is taken, the field will be diluted, training will remain splintered, and program efficacy will be hampered. The new model should be empirically-based and have the capacity to encourage flexibility and linkages across the entire treatment/rehabilitation system. A comprehensive treatment/rehabilitation model would reharness the energies of the current existing tandem systems in order to make them parallel, more interactive, and eventually integrated.

ACKNOWLEDGEMENTS

This chapter represents an early version of a paper published by the Journal of Nervous and Mental Disease 1987, 175 (6):317–326. This research was supported with funds from NIMH Grants No. 29575, 40607, 34365, and 00340. In addition, the authors would like to express their appreciation to members of the Rehabilitation Consortium of Greater New Haven, counselors and administrators of the New Haven and Central offices of the Connecticut Division of Vocational Rehabilitation, and the team directing the activities at the Boston University Center for Rehabilitation Research and Training in Mental Health for their time, patience, and expertise in educating us about their agencies and the processes involved in rehabilitation. The authors commend participants in this survey for their willingness to permit review, their frankness in interviews, and their high degree of problem-solving ingenuity. We also wish to thank Boris Astrachan, M.D.; Celia Brown; Marilyn Campbell, Ph.D.; Earl Giller, M.D.; Edward Ryan, Ph.D.; Morris Bell, Ph.D.; William Anthony, Ph.D.; Paul Parente, M.S.W.; Joseph Parente; and James Rascati, A.C.S.W. for manuscript review. The authors are also very grateful to Nancy Ryan at Yale and Ellen Rector at UCHSC for manuscript revisions.

REFERENCES

Adler, D.A. (1981) "The medical model and psychiatry's tasks", *Hosp. Community Psychiatry*, 32, 387–392.

Albee, G.W. (1969) "Emerging concepts of mental illness and models of treatment: The psychological point of view", *Am. J. Psychiatry*, 125, 870–876.

Anderson, C.M., Hogarty G.E. and Reiss, D.J. (1980) Family treatment of adult schizophrenic patients: a psycho–educational approach. *Schizophr. Bull.*, 6, 490–505.

Anthony, W.A. (1979a) *Principles of Psychiatric Rehabilitation*, Baltimore: University Park.

Anthony, W.A. (1979b) "The rehabilitation approach to diagnosis", *N. Directions Ment. Health Serv.* 2, 25–36.

Anthony, W.A. (1982) "Explaining "psychiatric rehabilitation" by an analogy to "physical rehabilitation", *Psychosoc. Rehabil. J.*, 5, 61–66.

Anthony, W.A. and Buell, G. (1973) "Psychiatric aftercare clinic effectiveness as a function of patient demographic characters", *J. Consult. Clin. Psychol.*, 41, 116–119.

Anthony, W.A., Cohen, M.R., and Vitalo, R. (1978) "The measurement of rehabilitation outcome", *Schizophr. Bull.*, 4, 365–383.

Anthony, W.A., Cohen, M.R., and Cohen, B.F. (1984) "Psychiatric rehabilitation", in: J.A. Talbott, (Ed.), *The Chronic Mental Patient*, New York: Grune & Stratton, 137–157.

Anthony, W.A., and Margules, A. (1974) "Toward improving the efficacy of psychiatric rehabilitation: a skills training approach", *Rehabil. Psychol.*, 21, 101–105.

Astrachan, B.M., Levinson, D.J., and Adler, D.A. (1976) "The impact of national health insurance on the tasks and practice of psychiatry", *Arch. Gen. Psychiatry*, 33, 785–794.

Bandura, A. and Walters, R.H. (1963) *Social Learning and Personality Development*, New York: Holt, Rinehardt, & Winston.

Beard, J.H., Propst, R.N., and Malamud, T.J. (1982) "The Fountain House model of psychiatric rehabilitation", *Psychosoc. Rehabil. J.*, 5, 47–53.

Berger, P. (Ed.) (1964) *The Human Shape of Work,* South Bend, IN: Gateway.

Bernheim, R. (1987) "Family consumerism: coping with the winds of change", in:, *Families of the Mentally Ill: Coping and Adaptation*, (Eds. A.Hatfield and H. Lefley), New York, Guilford

Black, B.J. (1976) "Rehabilitative and community support for mental patients", *Rehabil. Lit.*, 37(2), 34–40.

Blaney, P.H. (1975) "Implications of the medical model and its alternatives", *Am. J. Psychiatry*, 132(9):911–914.

Bleuler, M. (1972) *The Schizophrenic Disorders:Long–term Patient and Family Studies.* Translated by S.M. Clemens, New Haven, Yale University. (Original work published 1972).

Bond, E.D. (1947) *Dr. Kirkbride and His Mental Hospital*, Philadelphia, J.B. Lippincott.

Breier, A. and Strauss, J.S. (1983) "Self–control in psychiatric disorders", *Arch. Gen. Psychiatry*, 40(10), 1141–1145.

Breier, A. and Strauss, J.S. (1984) "Social relationships in the recovery from psychotic disorder", *Am. J. Psychiatry*, 141(8), 949–955.

Burke, D.A. and Sellin, D.F. (1972) "Measuring the self–concept of ability as a worker", *Except. Child*, October, 126–151.

Cheadle, A.J., Cushing, D., Drew, C.D.A. et al. (1967) "The measurement of the work performance of psychiatric patients", *Br. J. Psychiatry*, 113, 841–846.

Chittick, R.A., Brooks, G.W., Irons, F.A., and Deane, W.N. (1961) *The Vermont Story.* Burlington, VT, Queen City.

Ciompi, L. and Müller C. (1976) *The Life Course and Aging in Schizophrenia: A Catamnestic Llongitudinal Sstudy into Advanced Age*, Berlin, Springer/Verlag.

Clausen, J.A. (1975) "The impact of mental illness: a twenty–year follow–up", in *LifeHistoryResearch in Psychopathology*, (Eds. R.T. Wirt, G. Winokur, and M. Roff), Vol. IV, Minneapolis, MN, University of Minnesota.

Cohen, M. (1981) *Improving Intra-agency Collaboration Between Vocational Rehabilitation and Mental Health Agencies: A Conference Summary Report*, Boston, MA Center for Rehabilitation Research and Training in Mental Health.

Cole, N. and Shupe, D. (1970) "A four–year follow–up of former psychiatric patients in industry", *Arch. Gen. Psychiatry*, 22, 222–229.

Dellario, D.J. (1982) "On the evaluation of community–based alternative living arrangements (ALAs) for the psychiatrically disabled", *Psychosoc. Rehabil. J.*, 5(1), 35–39.

Dilling, H., Albrecht, J., and Deneux, R. (1973) "Investigation of performance evaluation and payment in the work therapy of chronic schizophrenics", *Soc. Psychiatry*, 8, 41–52.

Dincin, J. (1981) "A community agency model", in *The Chronically Mentally Ill*, (Ed J.A. Talbot), New York, Human Sciences Press, 212–226.

Disher, H. (1985). *Monitoring DVR in Montgomery County (MD)*, Bethesda, MD National Alliance for the Mentally Ill of Montgomery Co.

Dunnette, M.D. (ed.) (1976), *Handbook of Industrial and Organizational psychology* Chicago, Rand–McNally.

Early, D.F. (1973) "Industrial therapy organization 1966–1970", *Soc. Psychiatry*, 8, 109–116.

Engel, G.L. (1977) "The need for a new medical model: challenge for biomedicine" *Science*, Washington, DC, 196, 129–136.

Engel, G.L. (1980) "The clinical application of the bio–psychosocial model", *Am. J Psychiatry*, 137, 535–544.

Fairweather, G.W. et al. (1969) *CommunityLife for the MentallyIll*, Chicago, Aldine.

Freud, S. (1930/1953) "Civilization and its discontents", in *The Standard Edition of th Complete Psychological Works of Sigmund Freud*, (Ed. J. Strachey), 21, 64–145 (Original work published 1930.)

Griffiths, R.D.P. (1973) "A standardized assessment of the work behavior of psychiatri patients", *Br. J. Psychiatry*, 123, 403–408.

Grob, S. (1983) "Psychosocial rehabilitation centers: old wine in a new bottle" in *Th Chronic Psychiatric Patient in the Community* (Eds. I. Barofsky, and R. Budson) New York, SP Medical & Scientific, 265–280.

Harding, C.M., Brooks, G.W., Ashikaga, T. et al (1987a). "The Vermont longitudinal study of persons with severe mental illness I. Methodology, study sample, and overall current status", *Am J. Psychiatry*, 144(6), 718–726.

Harding, C.M., Brooks, G.W., Ashikaga, T. et al (1987b). "The Vermont longitudinal study: II. Long–term outcome of subjects who once met the criteria for DSM–II schizophrenia", *Am J. Psychiatry*, 144(6), 727–735.

Harding, C.M., Strauss, J.S. (1985) "The course of schizophrenia: An evolving concept", in *Controversies in schizophrenia*, (Ed. M. Alpert). New York, Guilford, 333–347.

Harding, C.M., Zubin, J., and Strauss, J.S. (1987c) "Chronicity in Schizophrenia: Fact, partial fact, or artifact?", *Hosp. Community Psychiatry*, 38, 477–486.

Hartlage, A. (1967) "Hospitals' and patients' views of industrial therapy", *Psychiatric Quarterly*, 41, 264–267.

Hendrick, I. (1943) "Work and the pleasure principle", *Psychoanalytic Quarterly*, 12, 311–329.

Huffine, C.L. and Clausen, J.A. (1979) "Madness and work: Short and long-term effects of mental illness on occupational careers", *Social Forces*, 57(4), 1049–1062.

Kraepelin, E. (1902) *Clinical Psychiatry: A Textbook for Students and Physicians*, 6th ed., translated by A.R. Diefendorf, New York, Macmillan.

Lamb, H.R. and Mackota, C. (1975) "Vocational rehabilitation counseling: a "second class" profession?", *J. Rehabil.*, 41(3), 21–23.

Lazare, A. (1973) "Hidden conceptual models in clinical psychiatry", *N. Engl. J. Med.*, 288(7), 345–351.

Liberman, R.P., Muesser, K.T., and Wallace, C.J. (1986) "Social skills training for schizophrenic individuals at risk for relapse", *Am. Jr. Psychiatry*, 143, 523–526.

Loeb, A., Kaufman, A.G., Silk–Gibran, E. et al. (1974) "Factors related to retention of employment for graduates of a psychiatric rehabilitation program", *Am. J. Community Psychol*, 2(2), 165–172.

Magee, J.T., Fleming, T.J., and Geletka, J.R. (1982) "The new wave in rehabilitation: projects with industry", *Am. Rehabil.*, 7(4), 21–23.

Menninger, E.A. (1942) "Work as sublimation", *Bull. Menninger Clin.*, 6(6), 169–182.

Mordock, J. and Feldman, R.C. (1969) "A cognitive process approach to evaluating vocational potential in the retarded and emotionally disturbed", *Rehabil. Counseling Bull.*, 12, 136–143.

National Alliance for the Mentally Ill (1984) *Five Years of Progress, 1979–1984*, Publication of the National Alliance for the Mentally Ill, Arlington, VA.

Paul, G. (1984) "Residential treatment programs and aftercare for the chronically institutionalized", in *The Chronically Mentally Ill: Research and Services*, (Ed. M. Mirabi), New York, SP Medical & Scientific.

Posner, B.Z. and Randolph, W.A. (1979) "Perceived situational moderators of the relationship between role ambiguity, job satisfaction, and effectiveness", *J. Soc. Psychol.*, 109, 237–244.

Rennie, T.A.C., Burling, T. and Woodward, L.E. (1950) *Vocational Rehabilitation of Psychiatric Patients*, London, Oxford University Press.

Rosenthal, S. (1978) "A clinical perspective of work organizations", *Psychiatr. Opinion*, 19–28.

Rusk, H.A. and Taylor, E.J. (1949) *"New Hope for the Handicapped: The Rehabilitation of the Disabled from Bed to Job"*, New York, Harper.

Ryan, E.R., Bell, M.D., and Metcalf, J.C. (1982) "The development of a rehabilitation psychology program for persons with schizophrenia: changes in the treatment environment", *Rehabil. Psychol*, 27(2), 67–85.

Stein, L. and Test, J.A. (1980) "Alternative to mental health treatment. I. Conceptual model treatment program and clinical evaluation", *Arch. Gen. Psychiatry*, 37, 392–412.

Strauss, J.S. (1982) *The Course of Psychiatric Disorder: A Model for Understanding and Treatment*, Hibbs Award Presentation, Annual Meeting of the American Psychiatric Association, New York.

Strauss, J.S. and Carpenter, W.T. Jr. (1974) ",Prediction of outcome in schizophrenia: II. Relationships between predictor and outcome variables: a report from the WHO International Pilot Study of Schizophrenia", *Arch. Gen. Psychiatry*, 31, 37–42.

Strauss, J.S. and Carpenter, W.T. Jr. (1977) "Prediction of outcome in schizophrenia. III. Five–year outcome and its predictors", *Arch. Gen. Psychiatry*, 34, 159–163.

Strauss, J.S. and Carpenter, W.T. Jr. (1981) *Schizophrenia*, New York, Plenum.

Strauss, J.S. and Chen, C.C. (1977) "Cross–cultural predictors of outcome in schizophrenia", presented at the 6th World Congress of Psychiatry, Honolulu.

Strauss, J.S., Hafez, H. Lieberman, P. et al. (1985) "The course of psychiatric disorder: III. Longitudinal principles", *Am. J. Psychiatry*, 142, 289–296.

Strauss, J.S., Harding, C.M., Hafez, H., et al. (1987) "The role of the patient in recovery from psychosis", in *Psychosocial Management of Schizophrenia*, (Eds. J.S. Strauss, W. Böker, H. Brenner),Toronto, Huber, 160–166.

Strauss, J.S., Harding, C.M., Silverman, M. (1988) "A conference report: Work as treatment for psychiatric disorder – A puzzle in pieces", in: *Vocational Rehabilitation for Persons with Prolonged MentalIllness*, (Eds. J. Ciardello, M. Bell), Baltimore, Johns Hopkins University Press.

Strauss, M.B. (ed.) (1968) "Familiar Medical Quotations", Boston, MA, Little, Brown, 563.

Thorndike, R.L. (1949) *Personnel selection: Test and measurement techniques.* New York, Wiley.

Tischler, G.L., Henisz, J.E., Myers, J.K., et al. (1975) "Utilization of mental health services", *Arch. Gen. Psychiatry*, 32, 411–415.

Tischler, G.L., Henisz, J.E., Myers, J.K., and Garrison, Y. (1972) "Catchmenting and the use of mental health services", *Arch. Gen. Psychiatry*, 27,389–392.

Tsuang, M.T., Woolson, R.F., and Fleming, J.A. (1979) "Long–term outcome of major psychoses: I. Schizophrenia and affective disorders compared with psychiatrically symptom–free surgical conditions", *Arch. Gen. Psychiatry*, 36, 1295–1301.

Vaughn, C.E. and Leff, J.P. (1976) "The influence of family and social factors on the course of psychiatric illness: a comparison of schizophrenic and depressed neurotic patients", *Br. J. Psychiatry*, 129, 125–137.

Walker, L.G. (1979) "The effect of some incentives on the work performances of psychiatric patients at a rehabilitation workshop", *Br. J. of Psychiatry*, 134,427–435.

White, R.W. (1959) "Motivation reconsidered: the concept of competence", *Psychol. Rev.*, 66(5), 297–333.

Zaleznik, A. (1965) "Interpersonal relations in organizations", in *Handbook of Organizations*, (Ed. J.G. March), Chicago, Rand–McNally.

4

THE PHENOMENOLOGY OF SCHIZOPHRENIA

L. James Sheldon

To Felix: For teaching me the difference

INTRODUCTION

Phenomenology has been used as a method of analysis and inquiry since the Renaissance, with the study of the signs and symptoms of psychiatric disease representing a later application. As medical technology was virtually absent in Europe during the eighteenth century, the time-honored clinical methods of investigation—the study of natural history paired with the phenomenological analysis of cross-sectional aspects of the clinical presentation—were the primary tools of research into the disorder which would later become known as schizophrenia.

The circumstances surrounding the modern investigation of schizophrenia in North America were quite different from the earlier situation in Europe, and different methods of investigation were used to study the disorder.

Bounded by contemporary dominance of psychoanalysis and the emerging method of the biological sciences, the North American research focus centered on the cross-sectional presentation of the disorder. The research method focused on symptom clusters, validation, and reliability of the cross-sectional presentation with an implicit underlying belief that the cross-sectional presentation was static over time. This change to the dominant North American approach of the method of research led to an abandonment of the European

Schizophrenia: Breaking Down the Barriers. Edited by S.G. Holliday, R.J. Ancill and G.W. MacEwan. © 1996 John Wiley & Sons Ltd

database in favor of a new and emerging North American data base. In the author's opinion, this change of method and subsequent designation of diagnostic categories closed the door on a sophisticated study of schizophrenia before the fundamental aspects of the disorder were understood. Furthermore, three critical errors arose from this action. The first critical error was the definition of the diagnostic entity in a manner causing discontinuity with the earlier literature. The second critical error was misidentification of the core symptoms of the disorder. The third critical error was a failure to recognize the resultant reduction in diagnostic precision. The cumulative effect of these errors would confound research efforts for many years.

The alienation of North American psychiatry from European theory and practice, in turn, led to serious flaws in a diagnostic system that was meant to be the heart of clinical and research practice. As North American psychiatry became preoccupied with a partial picture of this complex disorder, phenomenology fell into disuse and both the longitudinal identification and classification of phenomena were perceived as unimportant in the selection of treatment and unrelated to outcome. It was decades before the core symptoms would be re-established on the basis of a broad yet sound methodological approach.

Recent advances in pharmacology have provided a two stage impetus to rebalance the North American approach to understanding schizophrenia. In the first stage, typical neuroleptics demonstrated the ability to control the apparent core symptoms (hallucinations and delusions) of schizophrenia — but individuals did not return to premorbid levels of function. The second stage began with the recognition of positive and negative symptoms within schizophrenia and the possibility of first predicting then demonstrating a differential clinical outcome based on the longitudinal nature of the phenomena of the disease and the use of typical or atypical neuroleptics. The robust clinical finding could not be ignored and therefore had to be accommodated within theoretical models. This, in turn, led to a return of North American psychiatric thought to the earlier European concepts.

The preceding arguments can best be demonstrated in the context of a historical overview. The chapter will commence with a review of early European literature and then address one landmark international study. It will then turn to a review of the North American concepts and conclude with some views on new challenges and potential future directions in the phenomenology of schizophrenia.

EARLY EUROPEAN INFLUENCES

While many clinicians consider the recognition of positive and negative symptoms to be a North American achievement, a number of European authors foreshadowed these ideas. In fact, almost every element of the constellation of positive and negative symptoms can be found somewhere in the pre-1950 clinical psychiatric literature. However, it is clear that the various elements recognized in the literature were not formulated as either a symptom complex or as relatively distinct symptom clusters until the 1970s.

For centuries practitioners have distinguished between the congenital presence of subnormal mental capacities and the acquired loss of mental capacities (Dufour 1770). For instance, Dufour examined the issue in 1770 and offered a classification of acquired mental insufficiency based on age. Onset in infancy was termed *betise*, onset at the age of reason was *imbecility* and in old age was *dotage*. Dufour's work was influential and provided a background against which premature cognitive decline, including that associated with psychotic states, was viewed.

Other authors have examined the origins, meaning, and mechanisms of delusional thoughts (Locke, 1793). Locke foreshadowed the current concept of delusions as early as 1690, noting that,

> "having joined ... ideas wrongly, they mistake them for truths,
> and they ... argue right from wrong principles." (Locke, 1793)

Even today, and allowing for the differentiation of ideas from language, Locke's ideas remain relevant. In fact, both of the principle elements of the current North American concept of a delusion are represented in his ideas. The first element, that a delusional belief is markedly inconsistent with experience, age and culture, is represented in the first portion of the quote. The second element, that the belief is firmly held, is represented in the second part.

Leuret advanced a parallel argument regarding the disturbances of thought form in 1834:

> *" ... ideas, deprived of a regular association ... give rise to the*
> *most unsuitable formations. Sometimes it is a natural bond,*
> *which enfeebled or damaged ... sometimes it is a new bond*
> *that forms ..." (Leuret 1834).*

To the author, Leuret's work marks a step forward, as seen in the differentiation of the mechanism of association of ideas in health which give rise to normal thought form, as distinct from the altered association mechanisms in disease which give rise to improper thought form. There is also a strong parallel between Locke's concept of "joining" with Leuret's concept of association. The proper analysis of this similarity of ideas can be found in the concepts of meaning and meaningful connections advanced in the mid-1900's. Further analysis in this direction is clearly outside the scope of this chapter.

DEMENTIA PRAECOX

"Demence precoce" was a commonly used clinical term of the nineteenth century which was applied to any clinical condition, psychiatric or somatic, manifesting premature deterioration of mental abilities. Morel published a case report in 1860 of a 12 or 14 year old male which foreshadowed the current concept of cognitive deterioration associated with schizophrenia. It was not the first report of this clinical feature nor was it a formulation of a clinical syndrome (Morel, 1860).

His report described the dominant clinical feature of the case as the development of a violent hatred toward the father. Positive family history included a mother who suffered psychosis and a grandmother who was extremely eccentric. The once brilliant boy demonstrated intellectual decline over the course of his illness. Morel commented on the "sad termination of hereditary insanity."

The formulation of dementia praecox as a *clinical syndrome* is properly credited to Kraepelin (1899). It is critical to distinguish between the common clinical sign known as dementia precoce, which is described above, from the dementia praecox syndrome which was unrecognized prior to its formulation by Kraepelin.

Kraepelin drew the term from the observations of Pick, who had studied patients suffering from cognitive deterioration secondary to neurodegenerative disorders, and from the observations of Morel who had studied cognitive deterioration secondary to alcohol consumption. However, Kraepelin revised the definition of the term, which previously had been based on a simple observation made in any one of a number of clinical disease states, to a constellation of signs and symptoms associated with a consistent natural history of a single clinical disease state.

Kraepelin foreshadowed the North American recognition of negative symptoms by more than seventy years. He described fundamental symptoms which approximate substantial elements of the negative elements of the Positive and Negative Symptom Scale. The three fundamental symptoms he described were: Impairment of voluntary attention, progressive deterioration of the emotional life, and disappearance of voluntary activity. *None of his fundamental symptoms relate to current positive symptoms.*

In the view of many psychiatric clinicians, only half of the symptoms held as constituting the 1990's concept of schizophrenia were identified at this time. To a smaller number of contemporary psychiatric clinicians, the core features of schizophrenia had been fully and completely identified in Kraepelin's work.

Eugen Bleuler took the construct of dementia praecox in a dramatically different direction compared with the work of Kraeplin (Bleuler, 1950). He coined the term schizophrenia to reflect the disturbance of the mind which he described in great detail in his book. Where Kraepelin sought to understand the natural history of the clinical disorder and validate the concept in that manner, Bleuler advanced the idea that certain cross-sectional features, when present, defined both the disorder and the expected outcome. In contemporary terms, Bleuler considered these symptoms both necessary and sufficient.

Bleuler completed his formulation of the disorder of schizophrenia by redefining the hierarchical symptoms first advanced by Kraepelin. The new *primary* symptoms were alterations of affect, association of ideas, and alteration of volition. All features of the disorder which would later come to be known as negative symptoms were designated as *secondary* symptoms.

On careful review of the many clinical examples given in chapter three of Bleuler's book, the author has concluded that the clinical observations are indistinguishable from clinical observations made by the author in patients clearly suffering from bipolar disorder. The clarity of these diagnoses on which the author comments was based on longitudinal history, including both manic and depressed phases, longitudinal phenomena, and differential response to medication in both depressed and manic acute states as well as maintenance treatment.

Bleuler's work remained an important component in the contemporary European concept of schizophrenia until the empirical studies of Schneider (Schneider, 1959). The results themselves, and the misapplications in which they were employed, served to distort the European view of psychiatry by generating an inappropriate emphasis on the emergent positive phenomena of the disorder.

Schneider (1959) studied a group of individuals suffering from a psychotic state with a consensus diagnosis of schizophrenia which his peers considered valid. His intention was to describe common symptoms of the clinical state. To this end, he carefully interviewed a number of patients who were suffering from schizophrenia. The majority of symptoms reflected the subjective experience of altered perception or altered volition. He did not intend that the symptoms be considered pathognomonic for the disease state and specifically cautioned against the use of his work in this way.

However, this work, which was only intended to determine common symptoms, has been pressed into contemporary service as identifying symptoms possessing both high sensitivity and high specificity.

Random chance and a degree of medical misadventure would combine forces to indirectly produce a comprehensive and carefully considered textbook of phenomenology. Karl Jaspers was diagnosed as suffering an incurable and rapidly advancing fatal illness during the latter portion of his medical training. Accepting that his period of active practice would indeed be short he embarked upon an academic review of the body of literature related to phenomenology. Fortunately, the medical advice was inaccurate and he produced a massive text as well as several smaller works over many years before his eventual death.

In the author's opinion, the definitive classification of delusional states was written by Jaspers in 1963. He described three levels of pathology associated with beliefs held by one individual and not shared by others. The discriminating factors were not dependent on the content of the belief and were independent of how others might judge the content of the belief. It was wholly determined by the psychopathogical mechanism by which the belief arose. In this way delusions proper, delusion-like ideas, and over-valued ideas could be distinguished.

In the author's opinion, the work of Jasper deserves careful evaluation as it offers specific clinical advantages. The first is that each individual can act as their own control by examining their premorbid decision making. Secondly, the determination that a delusion exists becomes relatively free of the examiner's own cultural experience and allows more objective transcendence of any cultural barrier that may exist between examiner and subject. The third major clinical advantage is the ability to objectively recognize and stage recovery from the delusional experience.

IMPORTANT INTERNATIONAL INFLUENCES

In 1973 the World Health Organization (WHO, 1973) conducted a study of schizophrenia in nine nations on several continents in both urban and rural settings. This study, which was called The International Pilot Study of Schizophrenia, examined the prevalence of schizophrenia, sensitivity of symptoms of schizophrenia, and specificity of symptoms of schizophrenia. The prevalence of schizophrenia was similar in all populations studied. The experience of auditory hallucinations was very common and it was the most sensitive symptom of schizophrenia as well. The experience of control of the self by external agencies was less common and it was the most specific symptom of schizophrenia.

The author believes this was an important study. The size of the study offers reasonable statistical power. The great variety of environments and cultures studied speaks to both of validity and generalizability. The study confirmed Schneider's work when considered in the context he intended it to be used. It also raised the issue of two categories of first rank symptoms — those that are sensitive and those that are specific. Unfortunately this issue was not yet reflected in any diagnostic classification.

THE INITIAL NORTH AMERICAN EXPERIENCE

THEORETICAL DISCONTINUITY

North American and European phenomenological descriptions of schizophrenia were at the same moment unified and separated with the first edition of the Diagnostic and Statistical Manual (DSM) in 1952. The title of the DSM entity "Schizophrenic Reaction" bears a strong resemblance to the title of Eugen Bleuler's work "The Schizophrenias" (Bleuler, 1950). However, the manual drew from the work of Emil Kraepelin to define the diagnostic entity, with the DSM explicitly stating that the schizophrenic reaction was synonymous with the concept of dementia praecox. Yet, in the following paragraphs, the disturbances of mental life described as constituting the reaction were not those designated by Kraepelin as constituting the syndrome of dementia praecox. In the author's opinion, the phenomena described in DSM were more compatible with the findings of Bleuler. In retrospect, it appears that Bleuler's formulation of schizophrenia was more compatible with the emerging North American research focus and method than was the work of Kraepelin. Thus, an enduring discontinuity between the European and North American schools of thought regarding schizophrenia was established. This discontinuity would remain until the publication of DSM-III-R.

MISIDENTIFICATION OF CORE SYMPTOMS

By definition,   the DSM diagnosis of schizophrenia was established by determining the point presence of firstly fundamental and secondarily associated disturbances of mental life. Disturbances of reality relationships and disturbances of concept formation were designated as the two fundamental disturbances. Disturbances in affect and intellect were designated as associated disturbances. This distinction roughly captures what are now considered to be positive and negative symptoms.

The idea that emergent abnormal phenomena are associated with the diagnosis of schizophrenia had entered the English medical literature in a dramatic fashion in 1950 with the translation of Bleuler's work "Das Schizophrenias". Bleuler's work was well received and generated considerable interest among North American psychiatrists. However, Bleuler's emergent mental phenomena represented only one aspect of the established European view of schizophrenia. And, unfortunately, Bleuler's analysis was not accompanied by an analysis of the continuity of the work with the preceding literature. As has been explained earlier in the chapter, the historically earlier work of Kraepelin was the culmination of other authors' even earlier work which had been solidified and validated by longitudinal analysis of the cases forming the argument. Schneider's work, which was done after Kraepelin's and was the first substantial work systematically investigating emergent abnormal psychic phenomena, was not a longitudinal analysis. It was a cross-sectional evaluation with limited application which the author himself cautioned could be misused by the uninformed. Bleuler's analysis was based again on cross-sectional analysis of clinical cases but no such caution was offered. Bleuler, in point of fact, drew firm conclusions from his data.

Thus relatively unconfirmed findings formed some basis for the designation of the fundamental disturbances of schizophrenia. With the subsequent benefit of broad clinical experience, most clinicians would later agree that these emergent, or as now considered positive, symptoms were not restricted to the disease of schizophrenia and could be seen in many other psychiatric and somatic disorders. Curiously, those disturbances designated as secondary disturbances in DSM closely approximated the disturbances which Kraepelin considered fundamental.

DIAGNOSTIC PRECISION

Another enduring, and less well understood, difference between North American and European psychiatry was established by the DSM. This difference would adversely impact on diagnostic precision for many years.

The DSM clearly advocated the position that a morbid aberration of mental life, such as those seen in schizophrenia, should be viewed as a disturbance rather than as a phenomenon. As this occurred, the North American definition of signs and symptoms of the disease became discontinuous with established European literature. Although North American psychiatry remained preoccupied with phenomena (i.e. the observable unusual symptoms or signs of schizophrenia), phenomenology as a method of clinical investigation, with its tradition of long-term detailed analysis, came to be seen as irrelevant. In fact, clinicians quickly realized that the DSM categories were by no means complete and sought to alter the DSM by providing a glossary of definitions in subsequent editions of the DSM. These definitions, formulated largely with the cross-sectional method of study, lacked the fine distinctions and refinement found in the established European phenomenologic literature.

In short, the thrust of the DSM was to base the diagnosis of schizophrenia by the cross-sectional presence of disturbances of mental life which met *specific criteria* rather than on the longitudinal presence of *specific phenomena*. However, the criteria were relatively new, relatively untried, and without established validity. Further, the longitudinal presence and longitudinal nature of the criteria were neither established nor required. In terms of the downstream implications for diagnosis, these activities ultimately led to a diagnostic structure with a high degree of sensitivity and a low degree of specificity. In the author's opinion, true positive diagnoses on the basis of this construct would be confounded by the inclusion of false positives and exclusion of false negative diagnoses as well. This confound would have unwanted consequences in subsequent clinical practice and research efforts.

Six of the subtypes established in DSM were constructed with similar reliance on the cross-sectional presence of disturbances of mental life. These subtypes were determined by the dominant symptom and therefore by the manifest content of the belief rather than the underlying mechanism of the disturbance. Both clinical experience and the phenomenological method speak against the content of the symptom as a stable feature of psychotic diseases.

However, in three further subtypes the designation was determined by the historical pattern of the disease. This method of diagnosis — initially by cross sectional features and then subtyping by natural history — would bring the most troubling confound of all. The initial group would consist of both true and false positive diagnoses, but both groups would be longitudinally stable. This would remove the fundamental differentiation between those appropriately included and those inappropriately included.

This state of affairs set the stage for research into an unstable entity defined by high sensitivity and low specificity. Thus, clinicians and researchers alike would commit diagnostic errors characterized by high true positive findings, relatively high false positive findings and lower but still significant false negative findings. The expected outcome of this exercise would be a heterogeneous cohort and a less than stable diagnostic entity composed of six less well defined and relatively unstable subtypes and three better defined and relatively stable subtypes.

The clinical experience with the paranoid subtype of schizophrenia is an excellent example of the difficulties that can arise from this type of diagnostic error.

On one hand, the longitudinal clinical experience with the false positive diagnostic group schizophrenia demonstrated a population with heterogeneous outcome. The subtype then consisted of individuals with similar cross-sectional presentations who would then have dissimilar longitudinal courses, either as a result of dissimilar natural history of their affliction or dissimilar outcomes from a single treatment applied uniformly across a heterogeneous population of afflictions. For example, individuals with either cocaine or amphetamine intoxication could pass for the paranoid subtype of the schizophrenic reaction. Yet, even untreated, their disease state would resolve. As well, there was another subgroup of individuals who were free of drug intoxication who could present with cross-sectional symptoms indistinguishable from the paranoid subtype. These individuals would recover and return to their premorbid baseline level of function without intervention.

On the other hand, the longitudinal clinical experience with the true positive diagnostic group demonstrated a population within the paranoid subtype with a homogenous outcome—stable cross-sectional features leading to the recognition of a predictable longitudinal course. Clinical experience with this population showed a persistent clinical course beyond stability of the presenting, and therefore diagnostic, features. The affect of these individuals was preserved late into the course of the illness in distinction to other subtypes of schizophrenia. There was also a more robust relationship between selected biological treatments and reduction of symptoms

The undifferentiated subtype of the schizophrenic reaction was dealt the least favorable hand of all. The subtype was not defined by any specific disturbance. Rather, the defining characteristic of the subtype was a lack of defining cross sectional features. This subtype would then act as a residual category with low sensitivity, posses a high risk of false positive diagnosis, and be expected to represent a heterogeneous population. The only saving grace was the designation of acute undifferentiated and chronic undifferentiated subtypes. This uncertain state of affairs became clinically evident in the diagnostic confusion between schizophrenia, depression, dementia and eventually schizoaffective disorders over the course of the individual's life. Clarification of this diagnostic confusion would not come until the concepts of positive and negative schizophrenia were developed.

THE NORTH AMERICAN REVISION

The publication of DSM-II in 1968 marked a fundamental change in the North American concept of schizophrenia. Leading edge thought was beginning to see schizophrenia as a disorder in the classic medical sense rather than simply as a reaction. This change in the thought resulted in a new *clinical* focus on the natural history of the disease. This change justified application of the traditional analytic tools of clinical medicine—the examination of natural history, epidemiology, and intervention/outcome studies. Application of these tools to the study and treatment of schizophrenia would be shown to reduce the risk of false positive and false negative diagnosis and the DSM-II subtypes could be drawn from a potentially better defined and more stable diagnostic entity.

DSM-II redefined the fundamental disturbances that characterized the disorder with a new focus on changes in thought form and thought content. Clinical observations such as knight's move, loosening of associations and thought blocking were now part of a larger framework. Unfortunately, these gains would be more than offset by problems resulting from the relatively imprecise definitions of delusions and hallucinations offered by DSM-II. Changes in empathy, mood, and behavior were explicitly established as consequences of the fundamental disturbances. The ideas which would eventually develop into the concept of positive symptoms were now in place. Unfortunately, those features which would eventually form the basis of the negative symptoms were still viewed as epiphenomena.

DIAGNOSTIC PRECISION REVISITED

DSM-III (DSM, 1980) represented the most significant North American contribution to the quality of the diagnosis of schizophrenia. The issue of validity was expressly pursued by traditional methods proven effective in other areas of medicine. Familial patterns, onset, recurrence, and differential response to somatic therapy were identified as markers of validity. (These markers have consistently been demonstrated as valid tools in the investigation of other disease states.) Markers, however, are not the same as phenomenologic findings. In point of fact, phenomenologic findings are distinctly different from risk factors and risk markers.

DSM-III also spoke to the issue of natural history. Age at onset, deterioration of function, a psychotic active phase, characteristic symptoms, and minimum duration of the episode offered the clear potential of reduced false negative and reduced false positive diagnosis.

Further understanding of the nature of the disorder was seen in the assertion that symptoms were the result of alterations in multiple mental processes. This was an official embodiment of the growing literature reflecting the interconnectedness and the interdependence of each anatomical area of the brain. Perhaps the best clinical example is language. Impairments in the parietal, temporal and or frontal lobe will result in different forms of language impairment. DSM-III was an effective termination of the residual idea of one cause or one lesion resulting in a single and specific symptom.

The introduction of DSM-III-R (DSM, 1987) preserved the improvements made in DSM-III which had provided a better quality of diagnosis. However, ideas from Kurt Schneider were incorporated into the diagnostic criteria in a manner in which they were not intended by their originator. As a result, symptoms which can be experienced in other psychotic and somatic disorders could now result in a false positive diagnosis of schizophrenia. Unfortunately, when those symptoms occur in the other disorders, they often respond to neuroleptics. Thus, a very unfortunate stage was set in which symptoms weighted strongly enough to be on the verge of pathognomonic would promote a false positive diagnosis.

A common clinical example of this type of diagnostic misadventure is the mistaken diagnosis of bipolar disorder with auditory hallucinations as paranoid schizophrenia. The errant diagnosis would bring the clinician to prescribe neuroleptics in the expectation of an appropriate clinical response. The individual's now incorrectly diagnosed disorder would be treated in a less than optimal fashion but the symptoms would be reduced or even remit. The error in diagnosis would then not only go undetected but be incorrectly affirmed as all would appear well on the surface. The error would not be discovered until a review of the natural history of the disorder at a future date. In the author's clinical experience, this was often the case in bipolar presentations when alterations in thought content were prominent. A similar finding was made at a tertiary treatment center for treatment resistant schizophrenia (Smith et al., 1992).

Clinicians have long recognized both the appearance of new experiences in mental life and the loss of usual experiences of mental life as signs and symptoms associated with schizophrenia. A limited number of investigators made several attempts to clarify the nature of these symptoms and standardize the reporting of them. After several attempts, the concept of positive and negative symptoms was advanced in the late 1970s. A sophisticated and standardized rating instrument was designed by Kay et al., 1989, 1987) which was to serve as the springboard for rigorous evaluation of the response of negative symptoms to somatic therapies. This method of data collection and reporting coupled with the development of combined D2 and 5HT-2 antagonists led to dramatic changes in the North American concept of schizophrenia.

CORE SYMPTOMS RECONSIDERED

DSM-IV (DSM, 1994) addressed the issue of validity indirectly by employing criteria which effectively addressed the issue of natural history and almost as effectively addressed the issue of cross-sectional features. The frequency of false positive diagnosis and false negative diagnosis was therefore effectively addressed at a conceptual level. However, the potential for misdiagnosis remained by way of continued inclusion of Schneiderian criteria as an overweighted diagnostic criteria.

DSM-IV also represented the re-emergence of phenomenology as a pivotal element of the assessment of schizophrenia, albeit in an indirect way. In previous editions the diagnostic symptoms were derived from the glossary included within the text. The concept of positive and negative symptoms was incorporated into this edition.

As the concepts of negative symptoms, and to a lesser degree positive symptoms, were related to the traditional phenomenological literature rather than to the glossary, the symptoms in effect represented phenomennological concepts. The lack of refined analysis in the positive and negative symptoms, compared with that of the underlying phenomenological concepts, still served to limit the degree of diagnostic discrimination.

For some years prior to the introduction of DSM-IV, atypical antipsychotic agents were demonstrating a differential efficacy against positive and negative symptoms. Persistent clinical observations were made regarding the effectiveness of phenothiazine and butyrophenone derivatives against positive symptoms. Clinical observations were also made of the ineffectiveness of these somatic treatments against negative symptoms. The issue of neuroleptic induced dysphoria also arose from these clinical observations.

Negative symptoms would eventually succumb to somatic treatment. Clozapine, a member of an atypical class of medication, was shown to be an effective intervention in treatment resistant schizophrenia. This diagnostic entity is often dominated by positive symptoms. This atypical class was shown effective in schizophrenia dominated by negative symptoms as well. This was a clear difference in treatment outcome as well as emergent side effect profile compared with typical neuroleptics. Risperidone, another atypical neuroleptic, showed a differential effect against positive and negative symptoms on the basis of dose. Pharmacodynamic studies suggest a pharmacodynamic basis for this clinical observation. After almost two centuries of refinement, somatic treatments confirmed a clinical difference in treatment outcome based on the presenting phenomenology.

At this point North American psychiatry stands at the cross roads of schizophrenia. The linkage of new diagnostic descriptors to traditional phenomenological thought, by way of the Positive and Negative Syndrome Scale for Schizophrenics (PANSS) (Kay et al., 1985), has defined two subgroups of schizophrenia with sufficient validity and sensitivity to determine the most appropriate somatic treatment and to accurately predict the treatment outcome in the short term. This state of affairs represents only one road.

The natural or untreated sequence of developing signs and symptoms over the life of an individual suffering from schizophrenia has strongly suggested two subgroups of schizophrenia. Those individuals affected by what is currently known as positive symptoms show a longer survival and a better preservation of their intellectual ability than those suffering the condition currently known as negative symptoms. Those suffering negative symptoms have a shorter survival and their intellectual impairment is both more severe and more rapid. This longitudinal journey represents the second and crossing road.

The implications of the cross roads are clear. Which direction will North American psychiatry take?

IMPLICATIONS AND CONCLUSIONS

The current state of knowledge regarding the phenomenology of schizophrenia is the result of clinical practice. Clinical practice is the avenue by which chance observations are made then later confirmed by others or with different clinical cases. Although deep thinkers have originated many of the current concepts, in general, these concepts have been validated and become generally accepted through wide application in clinical practice. It follows that phenomenology should be more widely taught and more widely used in clinical practice. It should not be used in isolation from other clinical skills.

Persistent attention to the natural history of schizophrenia has resulted in an improved understanding of the nature and the prognosis of the disorder as well as its subtypes. Once this was understood, the risks and benefits of different types of treatment could be assessed. The result of this approach was every clinician's dream—the concept of symptom clusters—positive and negative symptoms—and differential treatment responses to specific somatic interventions.

In the author's opinion, the future of phenomenology in schizophrenia rests with the study of the natural history of the relevant phenomena. At present, phenomena are assessed only on a cross-sectional basis rather than a longitudinal basis. In a parallel argument, the phenomenological method is at a stage reminiscent of DSM-II. It has not undergone any of the qualitative improvements associated with DSM-III, DSM-III-R or DSM-IV.

The current all or none concept of a delusion is the biggest single factor preventing improved clinical use of phenomenology. The individual trees of the forest appear as a blur of green through the current North American models of delusion. The blur of green is either present or it is not. A spectrum model of the delusional experience is unlikely to provide sufficient discrimination for research purposes. Jasper's model represents the best available classification tool. An epigenetic model may well meet the future challenge of providing higher sensitivity and specificity.

The current state of knowledge regarding the complex clinical syndrome presently referred to as schizophrenia strongly suggests that the current diagnostic structure cannot be maintained. From an historical perspective, the greatest degree of progress in defining a valid and stable diagnostic entity has been made by combing the work of careful observers and thinkers. With the power of traditional longitudinal methods of medical enquiry at this point in time, traditional methods of enquiry have increasingly focused on the natural history of the disease but modern phenomenological studies have been rigidly limited to cross-sectional phenomena.

The author believes that the current diagnostic entity should be both divided into two distinct entities and investigated as two diseases. The first proposed disease would subsume all subtypes with dominant positive symptoms and reflect the alterations of volition described by Schneider. The second disease would reflect the original syndrome defined by Kraepelin and reflect largely negative symptoms. Each diagnostic entity should be further and separately investigated by all methods available with the focus being the differences and similarities of the longitudinal course of the two illnesses. This method of investigation would compare and contrast the two disease states as well as identify those individuals suffering both diseases as a comorbid presentation.

In conclusion, the author believes that future contributions of phenomenology to the analysis, understanding and management of schizophrenia will depend on five issues being addressed. First, the current disorder of schizophrenia must be separated into two distinct disorders. Second, phenomenology must be more widely taught and clinically utilized. Third, an epigenetic model must be developed and accepted. Fourth, the natural history of phenomena must be learned. Lastly, the natural history of the response of phenomena to treatment must be determined.

REFERENCES

Bleuler E. (1950) *The Schizophrenias.* Translated by J. Sinken, International Universities Press, New York.

Diagnostic and Statistical Manual of Mental Disorders (1952) American Psychiatric Association, Washington, DC.

Diagnostic and Statistical Manual of Mental Disorders, 2nd Edition (1968) American Psychiatric Association, Washington, DC.

Diagnostic and Statistical Manual of Mental Disorders, 3rd Edition (1980) American Psychiatric Association, Washington, DC.

Diagnostic and Statistical Manual of Mental Disorders, 3rd Edition (Revised) (1987), The American Psychiatric Association, Washington, DC.

Diagnostic and Statistical Manual of Mental Disorders, 4th Edition, (1994), American Psychiatric Association, Washington, DC.

Dufour, J.M. (1770) *Essai sur les Operations de l"Entendement Humaine et sur les Maladies*, Merlin, Amsterdam, 357.

Jaspers K. (1963) *General Psychopathology*, Translated by J. Hoening, M.W. Hamilton, Manchester University Press, Manchester.

Kay S.R., Fizbein A., Opler L.A. (1985) *The Positive and Negative Syndrome Scale for Schizophrenics (PANSS): Development and Standardization.*

Kraepelin, E. (1899) *Lehrbuch der Psychiatrie, Defendorff*, Macmillan, New York, 1904.

Locke J. (1793) *An Essay Concerning Human Understanding*, Volume 1, 140-141, T. Longman, London.

Leuret F. (1834) *Fragments Psychologique sur la Folie*, 4, Crochard, Paris.

Morel B.A. (1860) *Traite des Maladies Mentales*, 565-566, V. Masson, Paris.

Schneider K. (1959) *Clinical Psychopathology*, Translated by M.W. Hamilton, Grune & Stratton, London.

Smith G.N., MacEwan G.W., Ancill R.J., Honer W.F., Ehmann T. (1992) *Diagnostic Confusion in Treatment Refractory Psychotic Patients*, Proceedings, Meeting of the American Psychiatric Association.

World Health Organization (1973) *Report of the International Pilot Study of Schizophrenia*, World Health Organization, Geneva.

5

AGE OF ONSET OF SCHIZOPHRENIA IN MULTIPLY AFFECTED FAMILIES IS EARLY AND SHOWS NO SEX DIFFERENCE

C. Walsh, P. Asherson, P. Sham, D. Castle, J. Williams, C. Taylor, A. Clement, D. Watt, M. Sargeant, M. Owen, M. Gill, P. McGuffin and R.M. Murray

INTRODUCTION

The majority of patients with schizophrenia first become psychotic between late adolescence and the mid-thirties, although wide variations in age of onset have been noted since the time of Kraepelin (1919). One factor which has been repeatedly found to influence age of onset is gender. Studies consistently show that the age of onset in males is five to ten years earlier than in females (Loranger 1984; Lewine 1988). This is not thought to be due to differences in symptom reporting or help seeking behaviour (Hafner et al 1991). It is maintained in different cultures (Hambrecht et al 1992), for different definitions of onset and diagnosis, and when gender differences in population age structure are incorporated into the analysis (Riecher et al 1989; Castle et al 1993). Moreover, these sex differences appear to be specific to schizophrenia and do not apply to the other functional psychoses (Loranger & Levine 1978; Angermeyer & Kuhn 1988).

While compelling evidence exists for a genetic component in the aetiology of schizophrenia, twin studies suggest that environmental agents also operate (Gottesman & Shields 1982). It is possible that the relative contribution of genetic and environmental factors varies between cases, and that genes are more

Schizophrenia: Breaking Down the Barriers. Edited by S.G. Holliday, R.J. Ancill and G.W. MacEwan. © 1996 John Wiley & Sons Ltd

important in some forms of schizophrenia and less important in others (McGuffin et al 1987). This raises the possibility that age of onset may be genetically determined. While a number of studies suggest that a greater familial loading may be associated with earlier age of onset (e.g. Kendler and McClean, 1990), there has been little exploration of the effect of familial factors on sex differences in age of onset.

To explore this issue, we have examined age of onset of schizophrenia in males and females from multiply affected families; in such families the illness is assumed to be largely genetic in aetiology. For the purpose of comparison, we have also examined age of onset in an epidemiological sample, unselected for family history.

MATERIALS AND METHODS

FAMILIAL SAMPLE

Families with a high density of schizophrenia were collected at three centres: 1) Institute of Psychiatry, London; 2) University of Wales College of Medicine; 3) St. John's Hospital, Aylesbury, Buckinghamshire. All families had originally been identified for genetic linkage studies (McGuffin et al 1983; Andrew et al 1987; Gill et al 1993) and were selected on basis of having a minimum of two, living, first degree relatives suffering from schizophrenia or schizoaffective disorder. Many families were identified because of a high density of schizophrenia in a single sibship, designated the 'index' sibship. In those families where no clustering occurred in a particular sibship, 'index' status was allocated to the younger (two affected generations) or middle (three affected generations) sibship.

All available family members were assessed for evidence of lifetime psychopathology by trained clinicians using the Schedule for Affective Disorder and Schizophrenia—Lifetime Version (SADS-L) (Endicott & Spitzer 1978) or a lifetime version of the Present State Examination (PSE) (Wing et al 1974). Details of psychiatric morbidity were supplemented with history obtained from at least one informant and hospital case notes. Every effort was made to interview and assess all first degree relatives of index sibships (approximately 80% directly interviewed). Details of second and third degree family members were obtained by family history interview and, where possible, supplemented by personal interview and case note review if history was suggestive of psychopathology. In total, adequate data for diagnosis were available on 471 individuals (245 males, 226 females) from 63 families. The average age at assessment (± SD) was 41.1 (±17.2) years for males and 44.4 (±17.0) years for females. Full details of sample ascertainment, assessment and original iagnostic procedures for each of the centres are outlined in McGuffin et al 1983), Andrew et al (1987) and Gill et al (1993).

:PIDEMIOLOGICAL SAMPLE

)etails of this comparison sample have been described previously (Castle et al 991). Four hundred and seventy subjects with a diagnosis of non-affective, on-organic psychosis were systematically ascertained from the Camberwell :umulative Psychiatric Case Register (Wing & Hailey 1974). This provides a ecord of all individuals in a South London catchment area who had their first ontact with the psychiatric services between the years 1965 and 1984. All ubjects receiving a Register (ICD-9) diagnosis of schizophrenic, chizoaffective, paraphrenic or atypical psychosis for the first time were ncluded in the sample.

)IAGNOSES

n order to standardise diagnoses, the Operational Criteria (OPCRIT) Checklist or Psychotic Illness (McGuffin et al 1991) was completed for psychiatrically ill ndividuals in both samples. This checklist includes items detailing psychotic nd affective symptomatology and is scored by computer to generate diagnoses inder a number of operationalised systems. For the familial sample, all sources ·f information (completed interview schedules, informant histories, PSE yndrome checklists, prepared vignettes and hospital case notes) were used to omplete the OPCRIT checklists by two independent raters (CW & PA).)perationalised lifetime diagnoses were then generated using the 3.2 version of he OPCRIT program. Inter-rater reliability (CW & PA) was estimated on 20 est cases and kappa scores of 0.70, 0.68, 0.68 and 0.73 obtained for DSM-III-R American Psychiatric Association 1980), DSM-III-R (American Psychiatric \ssociation 1987), Research Diagnostic Criteria (Spitzer et al 1978) and ·eighner (Feighner et al 1972) diagnoses respectively.

·or the epidemiological sample, the OPCRIT checklist was completed from iospital case notes (see Castle et al. 1993) and operationalised diagnoses (for irst ever episode of psychosis) were generated.

nter-rater reliability between one clinician rating the familial cases (CW) and ·ne clinician rating the epidemiological cases (DC) was estimated on 20 test :ases. Kappa scores were 0.86, 0.88, 0.68, and 0.76 for DSM-III, DSM-III-R, ₹DC and Feighner diagnoses respectively.

ANALYSES

MEAN AGE OF ONSET AND FREQUENCY DISTRIBUTIONS

Age of onset was recorded in two ways: (1) age at first contact with the psychiatric services; (2) age at first admission to a psychiatric hospital or unit. Using operationalised criteria, the mean age at first admission was calculated and examined: (1) by sex and (2) for different definitions of onset. Using Research Diagnostic Criteria (RDC) for schizophrenia, the percentage frequency distributions for age of onset in males and females were compared within and between samples. The significance of any difference detected between the two samples or between males and females was assessed by Student's *t* test.

FERTILITY BIAS, CENSORING AND AGE STRUCTURE

In families identified by a high concentration of schizophrenia in a particular "index" sibship (Figure 1), the direct ancestors or "index" relatives (i.e., parents/grandparents) will, of necessity, be selected for having offspring.

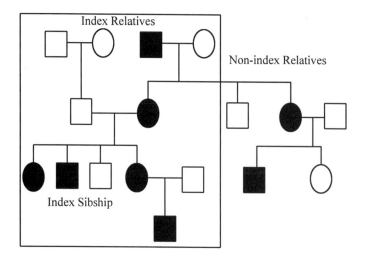

FIGURE 1.   Hypothetical Pedigree Illustrating Index and Non-index Relatives. Older Affected Index Relatives (generations I and II) Selected for Their Fertility

In contrast, "non-index" relatives (aunts/uncles/cousins) will be independently selected, irrespective of their fertility. Because female schizophrenics have a higher fertility rate, and because early onset of schizophrenia tends to preclude reproduction, a fertility bias will give rise to an excess of older onset females in upper generations. To determine whether a fertility bias was operating in the familial sample, the distribution and mean age of onset of males and females was examined, controlling for : (1) generation (older vs. younger) and (2) selection (index vs. non-index). Affected status was defined: (1) broadly (i.e. a clinical diagnosis of schizophrenia, schizoaffective disorder or unspecified functional psychosis) and (2) according to RDC criteria.

"Censoring" will tend to produce the opposite trend (i.e. a downward bias). Thus, family data will include young people who have not lived through their entire risk period (and who may yet develop schizophrenia), and information on other individuals may be missing beyond a certain age because of lost contact or lack of co-operation. To examine for the effects of censoring, age of onset (of affected subjects) and age at censoring (of unaffected subjects) were used in lifetable methods (the LIFETEST procedure of SAS 1985) to calculate a cumulative risk function. From the function it was possible to calculate the mean age of onset among all "susceptible" individuals, adjusting for censoring.

For the epidemiological sample, age distributions from the Office for Population Census and Surveys were used to calculate the annual rates of schizophrenia per 100,000 of the Camberwell population (method as described by Sturt et al 1984). The data were divided into four periods (1965–1969, 1970–1974, 1975–1979, 1980–1984) and age-band specific incidence rates were estimated for the different periods separately, together with their variances. These estimates were then combined into weighted averages; the weight of each estimate being the inverse of its variance. For the familial sample, calculations involved changing the denominator with increasing age so that, at any given age, the denominator consisted of those who had not developed the disorder and those who had not been censored. Thus, the denominator diminished with increasing age, and the effect was an inflation of the rate of illness in the older age groups. The annual rates of schizophrenia per 100,000 unaffected individuals in each age band were calculated using LIFETEST (SAS Institute 1985).

RESULTS

DIAGNOSES

In the familial sample, 190 individuals (99 males, 91 females) received a clinical, non-operationalised diagnosis of either schizophrenia (n=148), schizoaffective disorder (n=20), or unspecified psychosis (n=22). Of 63 families, 29 contained 2 affected individuals (first degree relatives), while the remaining 34 contained between 3 and 7 affected relatives. 128 of the affected individuals were contained in "index sibships", a further 27 were parents and 4 were offspring. The remaining 31 subjects were either second (n=14) or third (n=17) degree relatives. Complete data, including both OPCRIT ratings and age of onset data, were available for 142 subjects (75 males, 67 females), 92 of whom met RDC criteria for schizophrenia (49 males, 46 females). For individuals without complete data (n=58), the sex and generation distributions were examined and found to be similar to the rest of the sample. It is unlikely therefore that missing information presented a source of systematic bias.

For the epidemiological sample, OPCRIT and age of onset data were available for all 470 individuals, of whom 264 (132 males, 132 females) met RDC criteria for schizophrenia.

AGE OF ONSET

Table 1 shows the mean ages of first admission for schizophrenia by sex and for different diagnostic criteria. There was no significant difference in age of first admission for males and females in the familial sample (Table 1). This was in marked contrast to the epidemiological sample and applied for all sets of diagnostic criteria (Table 1) and for all definitions of onset (data not shown). Age at admission was notably earlier in the familial sample (24.53 ± 8.70 years vs. 40.46 ± 20.8 years); this difference was maintained for age at first contact (22.90 ± 9.19 vs. 40.07 ± 20.20).

Figures 2 and 3 show the percentage frequency distributions for age at admission in the familial and epidemiological samples (RDC criteria). Age at admission ranged from 15 to 66 years in the familial sample and from 16 to 90 years in the epidemiological sample. The distributions of age at admission in the familial sample were similar for both sexes. Compared with the epidemiological sample, age at admission of the familial group was shifted toward a younger age, particularly in females. A striking difference between the two samples was the relative lack of late onset cases in the familial group. In the epidemiological sample, the vast proportion of late onset cases was made up of females

Table 1. Mean Age of Onset for Males and Females in the Familial and Epidemiological Samples According to Different Diagnostic Criteria (* significance of gender difference)

DIAGNOSTIC CRITERIA	FAMILIAL SAMPLE MEAN AGE OF ONSET (±SD)			EPIDEMIOLOGICAL SAMPLE MEAN AGE OF ONSET (±SD)		
	MALES	FEMALES	P*	MALES	FEMALES	P*
RDC	(n=49) 23.65 ± 8.06	(n=43) 25.53 ± 9.37	0.31	(n=132) 33.56 ± 16.07	(n=132) 47.36 ± 22.72	<0.00001
DSMIII	(n=47) 23.29 ± 5.60	(n=33) 23.60 ± 6.80	0.82	(n=93) 26.94 ± 7.44	(n=40) 30.25 ± 9.39	0.032
DSMIIIR	(n=47) 24.46 ± 8.76	(n=34) 23.35 ± 6.91	0.54	(n=87) 32.41 ± 15.82	(n=76) 51.39 ± 21.16	<0.00001
FEIGHNER	(n=47) 24.48 ± 8.81	(n=32) 25.13 ± 7.56	0.74	(n=112) 32.17 ± 14.42	(n=85) 48.80 ± 21.63	<0.00001

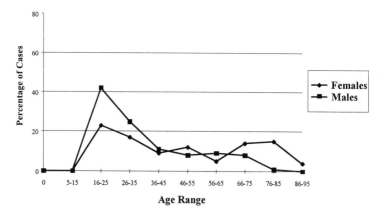

Figure 2. Age of Onset—Epidemiological Sample (First Admission)

Age Specific Incidence Rates

The annual age specific incidence rates for both samples are shown in Table 2. The numbers of affected individuals in each age band are also indicated.

Table 2. Number of Individuals Affected* by Family

Number Affected (n=90)	2	3	4	5	6	7
Number of Families (n=63)	29	17	10	3	2	2

* Affected status is broadly defined as a clinical diagnosis of schizophrenia, schizoaffective disorder or other unspecified functional psychosis.

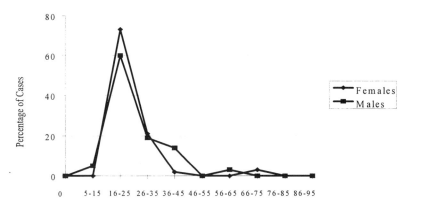

Figure 3. Age of Onset—Familial Sample (First Admission)

As expected, the incidence rates in the familial sample were considerably higher as these families were specifically selected for a high density of schizophrenia. Incidence rates were found to be similar for familial males and females in the same age band and there were few cases of either sex over the age of 45. In contrast, there were large differences between males and females in the epidemiological sample, with males showing much higher incidence rates in the younger age bands but females showing the highest rates in the older age bands.

CONTROLLING FOR FERTILITY BIAS AND CENSORING

Table 3 shows the numbers of affected (broad definition) and unaffected males and females according to generation (older vs. younger) and selection (index vs. non-index).

As predicted, there was an excess of affected females amongst older "inde'" relatives. Furthermore, age of first admission was significantly older in this group (Table 4), indicating a fertility bias.

Table 3. Familial Sample - Counts of affected and normal individuals in relation to sex, controlling for generation and selection[*].

GENERATION	SELECTION	SEX	NORMAL	AFFECTED
	INDEX	MALE	42	9
		FEMALE	37	20
OLDER				
	NON-INDEX	MALE	27	5
		FEMALE	16	7
	INDEX	MALE	63	73
		FEMALE	66	59
YOUNGER				
	NON-INDEX	MALE	12	12
		FEMALE	17	5

[*] Affected status is broadly defined as a clinical diagnosis of schizophrenia, schizoaffective disorder or other unspecified functional psychosis.

For all other groups, age of first admission was similar for men and women. These findings thus add weight to our initial results which did not control for fertility effects. With an adjustment for the effect of censoring on family data, the mean age at first admission was re-calculated. Using RDC criteria, the mean age of onset was 28.2 for males and 28.4 for females. This is older than that obtained prior to making the correction (23.65 ± 8.06 for males; 25.53 ± 9.37 for females), but still significantly younger than age of onset in the epidemiological sample.

Table 4. Familial Sample - Mean ages (with standard deviations) at first symptom, first contact, and first admission in relation to gender, controlling for generation and selection[*].

Generation	Selection	Sex	Mean Age at first symptom	Mean Age at first contact	Mean Age at first admission
Older	Index	Male	26.0 (12.4)	35.0 (18.6)	40.7 (12.6)
		Female	33.0 (11.5)	34.9 (12.5)	36.7 (6.6)
	Non-Index	Male	22.3 (11.5)	25.0 (4.6)	28.0 (7.1)
		Female	21.5 (2.9)	26.0 (5.6)	32.4 (9.7)
Younger	Index	Male	20.2 (6.5)	21.0 (6.9)	22.5 (5.9)
		Female	20.4 (6.4)	23.3 (11.1)	24.8 (9.7)
	Non-Index	Male	18.6 (5.0)	18.9 (4.4)	19.6 (3.1)
		Female	17.8 (6.8)	21.0 (11.5)	21.6 (7.3)

[*] Affected status is $\cong$ a clinical diagnosis of schizophrenia, schizoaffective disorder or other unspecified functional psychosis.

DISCUSSION

There were two main findings in this study. First, there was no sex difference in age of onset of schizophrenia in the familial sample. Second, age of onset in the multiplex families was significantly earlier than in the epidemiological sample.

Our findings are supported by existing data which suggest the absence of a sex effect on age of onset in multiplex families (DeLisi et al 1987; Wolyniec et al 1992; Leboyer et al 1992), and findings which indicate a trend towards a lower mean age of onset in "familial" as opposed to "sporadic" samples (Kendler and McClean 1990).

Previous attempts to characterise a genetic subtype of schizophrenia based on "familial"/"sporadic" distinctions (Baron et al 1982; Murray et al 1985; Owen et al 1988; Nimgaonkar et al 1988) have been criticised on the grounds that the rate of misclassification is likely to be high (Eaves et al 1986; Kendler 1988). However, in this study at least 34 families contained between three and seven affected individuals. This must greatly reduce the chance of false positives and lends some justification to the assumption that schizophrenia in these families is predominantly genetic in origin. Furthermore, this study did not attempt to identify a "sporadic" group. Instead, an epidemiological sample, unselected for family history, was used as a control with which to compare age of onset in the familial group. Indeed, approximately 7% of the epidemiological sample was documented as having a family history of psychiatric disorder and, if anything, this would tend to diminish any differences between the two samples.

Our epidemiological sample consisted of individuals in a defined catchment area who had their first ever psychiatric contact within a 20 year period. First psychiatric contact does not necessarily imply hospitalisation (20% of the sample were not admitted at first contact) and so individuals with relatively mild forms of the disorder as well as those with later ages of onset are more likely to have been included. Thus, in many respects, this sample may provide a more accurate representation of age of onset of schizophrenia in the general population. Moreover, even if this sample were in some way atypical, significant sex differences in age of onset have consistently been reported in other samples (Lewine 1988).

One explanation for our findings is that the disease in multiplex families is more likely to contain genetic subtypes of schizophrenia and as such, demonstrate a more uniform age of onset. Similar examples of this phenomenon have been described in other apparently non-mendelian genetic disorders such as

Alzheimer's disease, familial breast cancer, and non-insulin dependent diabetes (Goate et al 1989; Hall et al 1990; Bell et al 1991).

Alternatively, under a model of heterogeneity, sex differences in age of onset of schizophrenia in epidemiological samples could be explained if aetiological subtypes were to differ in their sex incidence. In this study, men and women from multiply affected families, assumed to share a common genetic aetiology, did not differ in age of onset. In contrast, there were marked differences in the epidemiological sample, with a preponderance of males in the under 45 age range and an excess of females thereafter. These data could be accounted for if a different mix of aetiological factors were operating in a late onset subtype of schizophrenia which is more common in females. This hypothesis is in keeping with data from other studies which also suggest that older onset females suffer from a distinct subtype of schizophrenia (Jones et al 1994).

Our findings could also be explained under a liability-threshold model of inheritance. This model proposes that the liability to develop schizophrenia is determined by both genes and environment (Gottesman & Shields 1967). While all individuals have some degree of liability (normally distributed), symptoms of schizophrenia will only emerge if this exceeds a critical threshold (Falconer 1965; Gottesman & Shields 1967). By specifying more than one threshold, the model can be modified to allow for different clinical forms of the disorder (Reich et al 1975).

Under a liability threshold model, sex differences in age of onset are expected if the threshold for being affected is higher in females than in males. This may occur because some factor associated with female gender protects against schizophrenia (e.g. anti-dopaminergic properties of oestrogens) and so more of the relevant genetic and environmental factors are required before females manifest the disorder. This is compatible with findings that the relatives of female probands are at greater risk of developing schizophrenia than the relatives of male probands (Pulver et al 1992; Sham et al 1994). Assuming a positive correlation between age of onset and genetic liability, the absence of a sex effect on age of onset in the multiplex families would suggest that the high gene dosage in females from these families was sufficient to override factors which normally confer protection. Similarly, the earlier age of onset in the familial sample as a whole would also be predicted by the greater familial loading. This is in keeping with other studies which suggest a positive correlation between age of onset and genetic liability.

It is apparent that our findings are compatible with a number of different models concerning the aetiology of schizophrenia and that, as yet, there is no strong reason to favour one particular model over another. However, it must be noted that both wide variations in age of onset, and sex differences in age of onset, are well established findings in epidemiological samples which clearly relate to the biological basis of schizophrenia. The recognition, therefore, that familial factors alter the usual pattern of presentation (as indicated by our findings) must represent an important avenue for further research into the aetiology of schizophrenia.

ACKNOWLEDGMENTS

We would like to thank all the families who generously gave their time to this project. We would also like to thank Dr. Biddie Andrew who collected data at St. John's Hospital, Aylesbury. This work was supported by the Stanley Foundation, SANE, the Medical Research Council, and by Wellcome Trust.

REFERENCES

American Psychiatric Association (1980). *Diagnostic and Statistical Manual of Mental Disorder, edn 3*: Washington, DC.

American Psychiatric Association (1987). *Diagnostic and Statistical Manual of Mental Disorder, end 3, revised*: Washington, DC.

Andrew B., Watt D.C., Gillespie C. and Chapel H. (1987). A study of genetic linkage in schizophrenia. *Psychological Medicine* 17, 363–370.

Angermeyer M.C. & Kuhn L. (1988). Gender differences in age at onset of schizophrenia: an overview. *European Archives of Psychiatry and Neurological Science* 237, 351–364.

Baron M., Greun R. and Asnis L. (1982). Schizophrenia: a comparative study of patients with and without family history. *British Journal of Psychiatry* 140, 516–517.

Bell G.I., Xiang K.S., Newman H.V., Wu S.–H., Wright L.G., Fajans S.S. and Cox N.J. (1991). Gene for non–insulin dependent diabetes (maturity onset diabetes of the young subtype) is linked to DNA polymorphisms on human chromosome 20q. *Proceedings of the National Academy of the Sciences USA* 88, 484–1488.

Castle D.J., Wessely S., Der G. and Murray R.M. (1991). The incidence of operationally defined schizophrenia in Camberwell, 1965 to 1984. *British Journal of Psychiatry* 159, 790–794.

Castle D.J., Wessely S. and Murray R.M. (1993). Sex and schizophrenia: effects of diagnostic stringency, and associations with premorbid variables. *British Journal of Psychiatry* In press.

DeLisi L.E., Goldin L.R., Maxwell E., Kazuba D.M. and Gershon E.S. (1987). Clinical features of illness in siblings with schizophrenia or schizoaffective disorder. *Archives of General Psychiatry* 44, 891–896.

Eaves L.J., Kendler K.S., Schulz S.C. (1986). The familial sporadic classification: its power for the resolution of genetic and environmental aetiological factors. *Journal of Psychiatric Research* 20, 115–130.

Endicott J. & Spitzer R.L. (1978). A diagnostic interview: the Schedule for Affective Disorders and Schizophrenia. *Archives of General Psychiatry* 35, 837–62.

Falconer D.S. (1965). The inheritance of liability to certain diseases, estimated from the incidence among relatives. *Annals of Human Genetics* 29, 51–75.

Feighner J.P., Robins E., Guze S.B., Woodruff R.A., Winokur G. and Munoz R. (1972). Diagnostic criteria for use in psychiatric research. *Archives of General Psychiatry* 26, 57–63.

Goate A.M., Haynes A.R., Owen M.J., Farrall M., James L.A., Lai L.Y., Mullen M.J., Roques P., Rosser M.N., Williamson R. and Hardy J.A. (1989). Predisposing locus for Alzheimer's disease on chromosome 21. *Lancet I,* 325–355.

Gill M., McGuffin P., Parfitt E., Mant R., Asherson P., Collier D., Vallada H., Powell J., Shaikh S., Taylor C., Sargeant M., Clements A., Nanko S., Takazawa N., Llewellyn D., Williams J., Whatley S., Murray R. and Owen M. (1993). A linkage study of schizophrenia with DNA markers from the long arm of chromosome 11. *Psychological Medicine* In press.

Gottesman I.I. & Shields J. (1967). A polygenic theory of schizophrenia. *Proceedings of the National Academy of Sciences* 58, 199–205.

Gottesman I.I. & Shields J. (1972). *Schizophrenia and Genetics: A Twin Study Vantage Point*. Academic Press Inc, Orlando, FL..

Gottesman I.I. & Shields J. (1982). *Schizophrenia – The Epigenetic Puzzle*. Cambridge University Press: Cambridge.

Hafner H., Riecher–Rossler A., Fatkenhauer B., Hambrecht M., Löffler W., an der Heiden W., Maurer K., Munk–Jorgensen P. and Strömgren E. (1991). Sex differences in schizophrenia. *Psychiatrica Fennica* 22, 123–156.

Hall J.M., Lee M.K., Newman B., Morrow J.E., Anderson L.A., Huey B. and King M.C. (1990). Linkage of early onset familial breast cancer to chromosome 17q21. *Science* 250, 1684–1689.

Hambrecht M., Maurer K. and Hafner H. (1992). Gender differences in schizophrenia in three cultures. *Social Psychiatry and Psychiatric Epidemiology* 27, 117–121.

Jones P., Bebbington P., Foerster A., Lewis S., Murray R., Russell A., Sham P. and Toone B. (1994). Gender and the phenomenology of stringently defined schizophrenia. Submitted.

Kendler K.S. (1988). The sporadic v. familial classification given aetiological heterogeneity: II Power analyses. *Psychological Medicine* 18, 991–999.

Kendler K.S. & McClean C.J. (1990). Estimating familial effects on age at onset and liability to schizophrenia. I. Results of a large family study. *Genetic Epidemiology* 7, 409–417.

Kraepelin E. (1919). *Dementia Praecox and Paraphrenia*. Barclay RM (trans.), E & S Livingstone, Edinbrugh.

Leboyer M., Filteau M.-J., Jay M., Campion D., Rochet T., D'Amato T., Feingold J., Des Lauriers A. and Widlöcher D. (1992). No gender effect on age of onset in familial schizophrenia? Letter to *American Journal of Psychiatry* 149, 10:1409.

Lewine R.J. (1988). *In Handbook of Schizophrenia* (ed. H.A. Nasrallah), Vol.3, pp. 379–397. Elsevier, Amsterdam.

Loranger A.W. and Levine P.M. (1978). Age at onset in bipolar illness. *Archives of General Psychiatry* 35, 1345–1348.

Loranger A.W. (1984). Sex differences in age at onset of schizophrenia. *Archives of General Psychiatry* 41, 157–161.

McGuffin P., Festenstein H. and Murray R. (1983). A family study of HLA antigens and other genetic markers in schizophrenia. *Psychological Medicine* 13, 31–43.

McGuffin P., Farmer A., Gottesman I.I. (1987). Is there really a split in schizophrenia? *British Journal of Psychiatry* 150, 581–592.

McGuffin P., Farmer A.E. and Harvey I. (1991). A polydiagnostic application of operational criteria in psychotic illness: development and reliability of the OPCRIT system. *Archives of General Psychiatry* 48, 764–770.

Murray R.M., Lewis S.W. and Reveley A.M. (1985). Towards an aetiological classification of schizophrenia. *Lancet i* 1023–1026.

Nimgaonkar V.L., Wessely S., Tune L.E. and R.M. Murray (1988). Response to drugs in schizophrenia: the influence of family history, obstetric complications and ventricular enlargement. *British Journal of Psychiatry* 18, 583–592.

Owen M.J., Lewis S.W. and Murray R.M. (1988). Obstetric complications and cerebral abnormalities in schizophrenia. *Psychological Medicine* 18, 331–340.

Pulver A.E., Liang K.L., Brown H.C., Wolyniec P.S., McGrath J.A., Adler L., Tam D., Carpenter W.T. and Childs B. (1992). Risk factors in schizophrenia. *British Journal of Psychiatry* 160, 65–71.

Reich T., Cloninger C.R. & Guze S.B. (1975). The multifactorial model of disease transmission. *British Journal of Psychiatry* 127, 1–10.

Riecher A., Maurer K., Loffler W., Fatkenheuer B., an der Heiden W., Hafner H. (1989). Schizophrenia—a disease of young single males ? *European Archives of Psychiatry and Neurological Sciences* 239, 210–212.

SAS Institute (1985). *SAS User's Guide: Statistics, edn 5.* Cary, North Carolina.

Sham P., Jones P., Russell A., Gilvarry K., Bebbington P., Lewis S., Toone B. and Murray R.M. (1994). Age at onset, sex, and familial morbidity in schizophrenia: Report from the Camberwell Collaborative Psychosis Study. *British Journal of Psychiatry*, in press.

Spitzer R.L., Endicott J., Robins E. (1978). Research Diagnostic Criteria: rationale and reliability. *Archives of General Psychiatry* 35, 773–782.

Sturt E., Kumakura N. and Der G. (1984). How depressing life is—life–long morbidity risk for depressive disorder in the general population. *Journal of Affective Disorders* 7, 109–122.

Wing J.K., Cooper J.E. and Sartorius N. (1974). *The Measurement and Classification of Psychiatric Symptoms.* Cambridge University Press, Cambridge.

Wing J.K. and Hailey A.M. (1974). *Evaluating a Community Psychiatric Service: The Camberwell Register 1964–1971.* Oxford University Press, London.

Wolyniec P.S., Pulver A.E., McGrath J.A. and Tam D. (1992). Schizophrenia: gender and familial risk. *Journal of Psychiatric Research* 1, 17–28.

6

THE RELATIONSHIP WITH THE SCHIZOPHRENIC PATIENT—HOW IT'S CHANGING

J. Joel Jeffries

EARLIER CONCEPTS

It was Hippocrates who long ago identified the need to work collaboratively with the patient.

> "Life is short; art is long; opportunity fugitive; experience delusive; judgement difficult. It is the duty of the physician not only to do that which immediately belongs to him but likewise to secure the cooperation of the sick."

This is a lesson that has to be repeatedly relearned by medicine as a profession and each physician individually (Jeffries, 1995). It is easy to yield to the temptation of applying hopefully helpful interventions upon the patient rather than negotiating them with the patient. This is particularly true in the treatment of schizophrenia where patients have been seen as lacking the capacity to take responsibility for their own care.

In the last century psychiatrists were known as alienists and the mentally ill were seen as alien to the rest of society and treated with less respect. At a more benign level they were seen as children who were vulnerable individuals. Certainly the illness does impair decision making and patients are vulnerable and need a measure of protection, and there is a difficult path to tread between necessary and excessive dependency.

Schizophrenia: Breaking Down the Barriers. Edited by S.G. Holliday, R.J. Ancill and G.W. MacEwan. © 1996 John Wiley & Sons Ltd

There has also been a tendency to forget the teachings of Sullivan, who pointed out that more than anything else patients with schizophrenia are human beings like the rest of us (Sullivan, 1931). Giving persons with schizophrenia their rightful share of psychiatric service and social dignity has been a struggle that has ebbed and flowed. Forty years ago, the advent of the "open door policy" and the introduction of neuroleptics were steps forward. However, the preeminence, at least in North America, of psychoanalytic psychotherapy in psychiatric practice in the post-Second World War period, led to schizophrenics, who were not ideal psychoanalytic candidates, being treated as second class citizens. As before, they were abandoned. Indeed, there was a fear of the illness as evidenced by the reluctance to share the diagnosis with the patient (Jeffries, 1977). When I began teaching patients about their illness in 1973, this was seen as rather radical. One exception to this conservatism was Dr. Abe Hoffer, who, believing that he had an effective treatment in megavitamin therapy, actively taught patients about their illness (Hoffer and Osmond, 1974).

The predominant negative attitudes towards schizophrenia helped to heighten the inevitable trauma of having a serious mental illness, although when such a theory was promoted it was greeted with a great deal of scepticism. Only recently has there been renewed interest in the traumatic effects of the illness (McGorry, 1991).

NEW INFORMATION

It was previously widely believed that this illness was psychogenic and that it would therefore respond to psychotherapy. In reading the work of Sullivan, Fromm-Reichmann and others from that generation, one can be impressed by their sensitivity and caring about the psychotic individual, yet we now believe that they were quite wrong in searching for etiology in parental mismanagement (Sullivan, 1931; Fromm-Reichmann, 1954). Well into the neuroleptic era there were those who held on to this belief of family psychogenesis (McGlashan, 1983). Whether or not the theory is correct, the evidence is that psychotherapy was of limited usefulness when used that way (Drake and Sederer, 1986). We are now in an era of a new view of psychotherapy in which the emphasis is not on treating the primary disability of schizophrenia but on preventing secondary disability. In this new psychotherapy the focus should be the trauma of the illness. The patient and the therapist together face the devastating impact of the illness, grieve about the losses it provokes and look forward to developing a sense of mastery of the illness and hopefulness about the future (Jeffries, 1977).

This new psychotherapy cannot be done in isolation. It has to be done in the context of education. This starts very early in the psychosis with reality clarification, where the patient is taught about the symptoms of their illness and where the professional staff repeatedly point out to the patient what is real and what is not. As the patient recovers and enters a non-psychotic (or less psychotic) phase of the illness, the education can become more intense, so that the patient may learn about what precipitates the illness in their case, usually including non-compliance with neuroleptic treatment, as well as what they can expect from the use of neuroleptics and other treatment modalities. This should be done in an optimistic way, at all times trying to maintain the patient's autonomy and seeing the patient as a collaborator who brings their own significant and irreplaceable information to the healing process (Jeffries, 1977).

As the psychotherapy proceeds it is possible to get into quite intense feelings through empathic understanding of the effects the illness has had upon the person and through the facilitation of affective expression. Historically it was believed that expressing affect was likely to cause schizophrenic patients to relapse. It is now clear that this is patently untrue and the misunderstanding probably arose because when they did relapse it often resulted in serious affective dyscontrol. Cause and effect became confused.

There is little room in the management of schizophrenia for a distant or, even worse, distancing, stance. Therapists have to be real, behaving naturally and warmly and without fear that this will be misunderstood by the patient (Jeffries, 1992). The writings of patients make it clear that even when they are their most psychotic they are able to appreciate who is sensitive to their needs and caring about them, usually if not always (Bachrach, 1996).

Claims have been made for different types of psychotherapy. There is probably no one best approach. The right choice of therapy depends on the interests and skills of the therapist, the education, intellectual capacity and psychological make-up of the patient as well as the degree of recovery achieved.

Family therapy has become very controversial. Its very name implies that the family needs therapy. There is therefore an implication that the family somehow caused the illness or is somehow perpetuating it. Understandably, families resent this and it probably accounts for the high drop-out rates of family therapy even though the therapists may blame it on family psychopathology (Butterill and Paterson, 1996). What do families need? They certainly need the opportunity to share their information about the illness ("debriefing"), to be allowed to express their feelings about what has happened to them and to grieve about what has happened to their family and to their child; they too need empathic understanding and thoughtful education (Lam, 1991). How does this reflect on the patient? It now means that professionals, patients and families are working together as a team. There is no longer any excuse for family blaming or the extrusion of families from the treatment process. That is not to say that the families of persons with schizophrenia have no psychopathology. There is psychopathology in all families and it certainly will be accentuated by a tragic event like the occurrence of schizophrenia in a family member. The family members may certainly be helped by "therapy" but it should be emphasized that this in no way attributes the illness to them.

It used to be thought that persons with schizophrenia had no insight; this does occur but a much more important factor in their lack of knowledge about being ill is their use of denial; a denial that may be perfectly understandable when faced with the reality of having a psychotic illness. Through empathic understanding and direct, even empathic education this denial may be reduced or removed and further education take place.

We now know that this disease has a variety of courses and outcomes. There is much better understanding of the prodrome. This was a concept not even taught 30 years ago and yet now we know that it usually lasts a couple of years and can be more than eight years (Beiser et al., 1993). We know that some people have illnesses that remit easily while other illnesses resist treatment. What is most important is that this is an illness which usually ameliorates when people get into their forties, although some people do have persistent symptoms all their lives (Marengo et al., 1991). This is important to know in terms of system planning and also because it gives us a realistic hope for the future for the vast majority of patients.

There has been much interest in the concept of high EE, a high level of expressed emotion in the families of persons with schizophrenia, which was thought to trigger exacerbation and rehospitalization. Its clinical usefulness has turned out to be very limited (King et al., 1994). There is now more credence given to the alternative view, which is that the phenomena associated with high EE are to a great extent products of the psychopathology of the patient. These phenomena are therefore better understood by the concept of Family Burden, this being the factor that leads to further breakdown; this is not just a measure of patient psychopathology but of the family's capacity to deal with that psychopathology (Kuipers, 1993). Thus the patient is no longer seen as a passive recipient of family behaviors but rather as an active participant in a complex interaction which may be ameliorating or exacerbating for their illness.

The barriers between professionals and patients have to some extent broken down so that there is now greater acceptance of Sullivan's view of the essential human qualities of people with schizophrenia and therefore greater acceptance of the patients' role in their own treatment. Schizophrenia used to be thought of as an illness that damaged people in various ways simply by the impact of symptoms. For example, it used to be thought that schizophrenia produced social withdrawal as an intrinsic symptom. An alternative view was that schizophrenia somehow removed certain capacities so that there were deficit symptoms which included social withdrawal. Now we think of it as an illness that has symptoms and creates disability. Patients adapt to this disability in a variety of ways. Sometimes they do not do this well so that their adaptations may complicate their problems. A more modern view would say that while the previous interpretations may be correct for some patients, it might also be possible to think of this social withdrawal as being an adaptation by patients who, because they have a psychosis, are feeling socially inept, embarrassed about their illness, and afraid that others will look down upon them as they look down upon themselves.

SOCIETAL CHANGES

A number of changes in our society have led to differences in the way that professionals and schizophrenic patients relate. Each of these changes may have both positive and negative effects and I cannot review each of them in detail. They are all worthy of extensive study so that I will mention each of them with limited reference to possible effects.

A greater emphasis on a client-centred approach has led to the client-centred needs assessment, where there has been emphasis on having the patient express their own needs and develop their own goals and collaborate with their therapist in developing a remedial program to achieve these goals (Anthony and Nemec, 1984). This is a wonderful thing for patient autonomy but clinical experience has shown that the sicker patients may not have the capacity to use this approach.

Whereas we used to talk of people being "disabled" they are now thought of as "challenged" with the outcome that there is a greater emphasis on their taking care of themselves. For example, having moved from institutionalization to placement in the community where patients were often in large residences or hostels, there has been an attempt in many centers to have them placed in housing where they were helped to maintain as much autonomy as possible. More recently there has been some pressure to move from what is called "supportive housing" to what is now called "supported housing", with an emphasis on people having their own apartments where they are maintained even when quite ill, by the application of the necessary human resources to maintain them in their chosen environment. While this clearly has great appeal from the point of view of patient autonomy, it will likely turn out to be very expensive.

No longer are persons with schizophrenia told to avoid relationships which previously were thought to lead to psychosis. Certainly the break-up of a relationship will be distressing for someone with schizophrenia just as it is for everybody else. That distress may lead to an increase in anxiety and a breakthrough of symptoms. However, we have to balance against that the stabilizing effect of having a relationship, the improvement in quality of life that comes from having a close companion, so that overall now we accept that marriage can be very positive for many though not all persons with schizophrenia. They may need special counselling in regard to whether or not to have children, and if they have children about how to minimize the impact of their illness on their child's development.

In the past, families were kept at a distance from the treatment of schizophrenia. It was common to hear complaints of how they were not listened to and not given any information. In 1977 it was Bill Jeffries who pioneered the Ontario Friends of Schizophrenics which has grown into the Schizophrenia Society of Canada, a powerful lobby group for the care of schizophrenics and for research on schizophrenia. In the United States the National Association for the Mentally Ill (NAMI) has likewise had enormous impact.

A very recent phenomenon is that in detrmining at who are "mental health stakeholders" some patient advocacy groups have made the reasonable claim that they are the primary stakeholders because they are the "reason" for everybody's involvement and therefore they should be the "first among equals" (Whyte, 1995). It a view that, if widely accepted, will have a major impact on future system planning.

Some socio-cultural changes have been negative.

In the last quarter century feminism has been a major force for societal improvement. This has lead to intolerance of violence against women. This praiseworthy change may have contributed to "zero tolerance" of violence on the ward which is directed at female staff by male patients, so that aggressive patients may be summarily discharged or have criminal charges laid against them. They are seen as fully responsible for their actions even if severely psychotic.

Malpractice lawyers flourish. There has developed some fear of chemotherapy because of the risk of tardive dyskinesia and fear of being sued. This has contributed to the trend towards low dose therapy (Baldessarini et al., 1995). Supporters of the low dose approach believe that this protects many patients from over-treatment with the consequences of both short-term and long-term side-effects and increased non-compliance because of these unpleasant effects. Against this is clinical experience, including my own, which demonstrates that many patients are now being undertreated and given less than optimal neuroleptic doses (Clements, 1996).

We are in a time of great fiscal stringency where governments are reducing the amount of money they spend on health care. The number of available psychiatric beds is dropping so that in many areas, including my own, it is now very difficult indeed to find a bed for an acutely ill patient. For this reason one has to be quite sick to be admitted. This means that many quite psychotic people, who in the past would have been hospitalized, are now walking the streets. The "homeless" include many persons with schizophrenia.

LEGISLATION

The legislation in regards to mental illness varies from country to country, state to state and province to province. However, there are certain trends that are significant. One is the quasi-judicial review of decisions to commit people involuntarily and impose treatment upon them against their will. In my province, Ontario, there are now review boards which will, at the patient's request, or after prolonged periods even without their request, review the treating physician's decision to keep the patient in hospital against their will. This is extremely costly in terms of dollars but it has certainly had the effect of creating more respect for patients' views.

With the rise of mental health consumerism there has been increased emphasis on the rights of the "consumer"/patient to have the last word on taking treatment. Consent to treatment legislation now makes it very clear that a paternalistic approach to treatment is no longer acceptable.

Associated with these changes is an increased emphasis on advocacy. Many psychiatric hospitals have resident advocates whose task is to alert patients to their rights and to facilitate their expression of these rights. Indeed, in Ontario an act was passed in recent years creating an office which employed advocates working in all branches of medicine. The dismay of the medical profession, fiscal stringency and a change of government has led to this legislation being revoked but the role of the advocates in provincial psychiatric hospitals remains. The idea that people would be paid to advocate for psychiatric patients has been anathema to many of the other stakeholders. Family members claimed that they were the true advocates for the patients; nurses did the same, as did physicians, and patients' rights groups.

DIFFERENT VIEWS

How do we now think of schizophrenia? In the past Foucault has compared it to leprosy, a disease which caused the sufferers to be extruded from society. "Lepers" were put into leper colonies and schizophrenics were put into large mental institutions in the countryside (Focault, 1961). Twenty years ago I compared this illness to cancer in that it was a disease that was so "unspeakable" that this diagnosis could not be shared with the patient (Jeffries, 1977). In recent years Oliver Sacks has pointed out to us a different way of looking at diseases. He explains how people with certain neurological disorders may have qualities that have adaptive value or at least make them uniquely interesting. Sacks would therefore talk about many such disorders as just different ways of being in the world (Sacks, 1995). This is not to say that they should not receive treatment but it does emphasize the individual value of each person no matter from what disease they suffer.

We remain aware that schizophrenia is a chronically disabling illness where victims need support despite the advent of various psychosocial approaches and new medications. The question that now faces us is who will and who can provide this support. A number of model programs have been developed which have a major ongoing commitment to persons with schizophrenia with the promise that they will have continuity. In practice this does not seem to happen. Either the program ends or there is major staff turnover. Until recently I was involved in a program called the Continuing Care Division which committed itself to ongoing care for a cohort of people with chronic mental illness. Using case managers it fulfilled its mandate very well but, when there were changes in personnel and financial cutbacks, the program was dissolved and the patients returned to the "community", to the chagrin of both the patients and the case managers. Continuity of care continues to receive much lip service but has limited reality.

Continuity of caregivers' is a great rarity. I now have patients whom I have been treating continuously for 27 years. This may appear good but while I am now thinking about retirement their illness persists. Families emphatically point out that in the end they seem to be the ones who remain continuously involved.
It has been complained that consumer/survivors are not being fully used as contributors to mental health systems (McCabe, et al., 1995) but the paradox is

that the term "survivors" has been defined as "freedom fighters who want liberation from the mental health system" (Everett, 1994). "Survivors" is a term that many professionals, including myself, find offensive. Yet I do agree that there is room for increased patient involvement in decision-making.

POTENTIAL NEGATIVES

It certainly has great appeal to think of patients as consumers who have a valuable input. However, it must be realized that there are potential problems with this. For example, a psychiatric hospital decided it would have consumers on its board. This decision became somewhat problematic when one of the board members relapsed into psychosis.

A psychiatric hospital decided that it would recruit patients as volunteers to support other patients. They chose patients who had been well stabilized on medication and who appeared to be doing well socially. Then the administration began to receive complaints from some of the patients who were being "helped" that the volunteer was sexually harassing them. Of course, this could happen with any volunteer and the organization would swiftly disengage themselves from the miscreant. It becomes very difficult to do this when the miscreant is a patient. Should the administration inform the patient's physician and should the physician confront the patient?

The newer legislation does not appreciate that sometimes patients really are seriously incompetent. We occasionally get into silly situations where there is some judicial or quasi-judicial hearing where the patient's lawyer is arguing forcibly for one of the patient's rights, and yet the patient is clearly incompetent to instruct counsel and getting their rights would lead to the risk of harm. The point is that some of the legal activity in respect of patient's rights is ludicrous and unnecessary.

It is wise to remember the lesson of the Bronx–Lincoln Mental Health Clinic that won a medal from the APA in 1965 but was dissolved in 1966, when the consumer-run board lifted the psychiatrists in their chairs and carried them out to the street because the psychiatrists refused to make their main focus the treatment of narcotic addicts. One of Toronto's most distinguished advocates for the mentally ill in the past twenty years recently found himself subject to legal action from disgruntled "consumers" carried away with their own power and their access to free legal aid.

POSSIBILITIES

Experience has taught me that attempts to forecast the future are difficult and expose one to future embarrassment. Nevertheless, the exercise is worth while if only to have us think about some possibilities. We are in a period of backlash against "advocates". In my province they have been driven out of the rest of medicine and it is possible that they may be driven out of psychiatry.

Because of the concern about the criminalization of the mentally ill and the neglect of the homeless mentally ill, there has been increasing pressure for compulsory treatment. The New South Wales Mental Health Act of 1990 included compulsory community treatment and a review of the effects of that legislation shows that two-thirds of people affected had schizophrenia and that the outcome was that they had increased treatment contact, with better compliance, decreased family burden and increased personal well-being. Similar legislation was passed in Saskatchewan in 1993 and compulsory treatment may become part of our routine practice (King et al., 1994).

Last year the Ontario Friends of Schizophrenics (OFS) made a position statement in which they suggested changes to the Ontario Mental Health Act. They wanted to delete the word "imminent" from the Act so that patients might be hospitalized without having to be at death's door. They wanted to recognize "suffering or deterioration" as well as the risk of physical harm as indications for involuntary hospitalization and they supported out-patient treatment orders. They want the severely mentally ill represented on planning bodies. If people offer "alternative treatment" for the severely mentally ill they wish to ensure that the alternatives are held to the same standards as are generally expected in medical treatment. They asked for a halt in bed reductions, more psychiatrists, speedy transfer of records and more education of G.P.s and E.R. staff about schizophrenia. They have also advocated for better education of the police. In regards to community services the OFS supported case management and supportive housing and called for more mobile crisis intervention. They requested that the move towards community care be kept on hold until there was adequate funding to make it feasible.

I fear the introduction of "managed care" to Canada. Early evidence for the U.S.A. is that in the search for cost-efficiency the provision of service for the seriously mentally ill may be pared down below appropriate levels (Geller, 1995).

CONCLUSION

So now the person with schizophrenia is treated with more respect and indeed has greater responsibility to become a more active participant in their own care. Families are no longer scapegoated but seen as essential contributors to the well-being of their sick offspring. Professional staff need to think of themselves not just as healers, but as educators and system organizers. In the future we should be striving for, even though we may never achieve, a seamless team, that includes all the stake-holders.

ACKNOWLEDGEMENTS

Special thanks to Ms. Patti Greenlee

REFERENCES

Anthony, W.A., and Nemec, P.B. (1984) "Psychiatric Rehabilitation." In *Schizophrenia: Treatment, Management, and Rehabilitation* (ed. Bellack, A.S). Grune and Stratton, Orlando, 384–389.

Bachrach, L. (1996) " What do patients say about program planning".In *Mental Illness in the Family: Issues and Trends*. (eds Abosh, B., and Collins, A.) University of Toronto Press, 13–46.

Baldessarini, R.J., Kando, J., and Centorrino, F. (1995) "Hospital Use of Antipsychotic Agents in 1989 and 1993", *Am.J.Psych.* , 152: 1038–1044.

Beiser, M., Erikson, D., Fleming, J.A.E., and Iacono, W.G. (1993) "Establishing the Onset of Psychotic Illness", *Am.J.Psych.*, 150: 1349–1354.

Butterill, D., Paterson, J. (1996) "Shifting Domains of Illness Management", in *Mental Illness in the Family,* Issues and Trends" (eds Abosh, B. and Collins, A.) University of Toronto Press, 84–104.

Clements, C. (1996) "The Brave New World of Patient as Business Unit", The Medical Post, Feb. 20, 36–37.

Drake, R.E., and Sederer, L.I. (1986) "Inpatient Psychosocial Treatment of Chronic Schizophrenia", *Hosp.Comm.Psy.*, 37: 897–901.

Everett, B. (1994). "Something is Happening", *J. Mind and Behav.*, 15: 1–2: 55–69.

Foucault, M. (1961) "Madness and Civilization", *Tavistock*, London.

Fromm–Reichmann, F. (1954) "Psychotherapy of schizophrenia", *Am.J. Psych* 111: 410–419.

Geller, J.L. (1995) "A biopsychosocial rationale for coerced community treatment in the management of schizophrenia", *Psych. Quarterly*, 66: 219–235.

Hoffer, A. and Osmond, H. (1974) "How to live with schizophrenia", *Citadel Press* Secaucus, NJ.

Jeffries, I.P. (1995) Editorial. *Int.Pediatrics*, 10:204.

Jeffries, J.J. (1992) "How to Talk to a Schizophrenic", *Issues in Schizophrenia,* Jan.

Jeffries, J.J. (1977) "The Trauma of Being Psychotic", *Can.Psy.Ass.J.,* 22: 199–206.

King, S., Lesage, A.D., and Lalonde, P. (1994) "*Psychiatrists' Ratings of Expressed Emotion*", *Can.J.Psy.* , 39: 358–360.

Kuipers, L. (1993) "Family Burden in Schizophrenia", *Soc.Psy. and Psych.Epid.*, 28 207–210.

Lam, D.H. (1991) "Psychosocial Family Intervention in Schizophrenia", *Psychol.Med.* 21: 423–441.

Marengo, J., Harrow, M., Sands, J., and Galloway, C. (1991) "European vs. U.S. Data on the Course of Schizophrenia", *Am.J.Psych.* 148: 606–611.

McCabe, S., and Unzicker, R.E. (1995) "Changing Roles of Consumer/Survivors in Maturing Mental Health Systems", in *Maturing Mental Health Systems: New Challenges and Opportunities* (eds. Stein, L.I., and Hollingsworth, E.J.), Jossey–Bass, San Francisco.

McGlashan, T.H. (1983) "*Intensive Individual Psychotherapy of Schizophrenia*" *Arch.Gen.Psych.*, 40: 909–920.

McGorry, P. (1991) "Negative symptoms and PTSD", *Austr. and New Zealand J. of Psy* 25, 12–13.

"Sacks, O. (1995) "An Anthropologist on Mars".

Sullivan, H.S. (1931) "The modified psychoanalytic treatment of schizophrenia", *Am. J Psych.,* 88: 519–540.

Whyte, J. (1995) Quoted in C.P.A. Bulletin, June, 13.

7

THE USE OF ANTIPSYCHOTIC MEDICATION: SOME ETHICAL CONSIDERATIONS

Barry D. Jones and Stephen G. Holliday

INTRODUCTION

The first antipsychotic drugs appeared in the early 1950s. Following the introduction of chlorpromazine a number of antipsychotic medications were developed and, for the first time in history, patients suffering from schizophrenia were offered treatments that could consistently lead to a decrease in the severity of their psychotic symptoms. As has been described elsewhere, the widespread use of first-generation antipsychotic agents led to the mass deinstitutionalization of mental patients in the 1960s and 1970s (Talbott, 1994). With an active treatment in hand and many patients returning to the community, the situation seemed to be going well. However, we now know that treatment and return to the community did not necessarily lead to dramatic improvements in the lives of persons suffering from schizophrenia. Not only did the first generation agents fail to impact on the negative (non-psychotic) features of schizophrenia, their long-term use was shown to increase the risk of serious extrapyramidal and motor side effects. While the overall situation was certainly an improvement over the past, the status quo achieved with these first generation anti-psychotic medication was an uncomfortable one for physicians and patients alike.

Although many new drugs were developed during the next decades, most were designed to produce a blockade of the dopamine (D2) receptor. This focus led to the development of medications that treated the positive (psychotic) symptoms of schizophrenia but had little impact on negative symptoms. And, in addition, the focus on dopamine blockade led to the development of drugs that produce

Schizophrenia: Breaking Down the Barriers. Edited by S.G. Holliday, R.J. Ancill and G.W. MacEwan. © 1996 John Wiley & Sons Ltd

dopamine down-regulation in the motor system and lead to such side effects as parkinsonism, dystonia, akathisia, and, with long-term use, tardive dyskinesia.

The medication situation in which the available treatments were only partially effective and associated with serious side effects was tolerated, albeit reluctantly, only because the alternative—no treatment—was less acceptable. Given the tragic consequences of schizophrenia to both the afflicted person and the family, the use of conventional antipsychotics, however risky, was deemed to be preferable to the almost certain alternative of a life of suffering and hopelessness.

The status quo began to change in the 1980s with the re-discovery of clozapine. Originally released in the early 1970s as a treatment for schizophrenia, clozapine was quickly removed from the marketplace following reports that its use was associated with the development of potentially lethal agranualocytosis. Despite the documented possibility of serious side effects, clozapine continued to be used in some European locations, justified on the grounds that it could treat schizophrenia in instances where other drugs had failed. Researchers also maintained that with clozapine significant therapeutic gains could be achieved without inducing motor side effects.

Accumulating evidence of clozapine's ability to produce significant therapeutic benefits while exhibiting a minimal side-effect profile led to a re-examination of its efficacy and safety. This resulted in a consensus opinion that clozapine could be an acceptable agent for treating patients who were refractory to treatment with conventional medication. In a representative study, Kane and his co-workers (1988) compared the efficacy and tolerability of clozapine and chlorpromazine in patients who had either failed to respond to conventional antipsychotic treatment or were intolerant of motor side effects. In this double-blind trial, clozapine was shown to be efficacious in the treatment of refractory schizophrenia. In fact, within six weeks approximately one third of patients had shown a clinically significant response to treatment with clozapine whereas a much smaller percentage demonstrated any improvement on chlorpromazine. Furthermore, extrapyramidal side effects (EPS) were seldom seen in those patients treated with clozapine.

Since then, researchers have demonstrated that long-term treatment with clozapine (up to one year) can lead to improvement in upwards of 50–60% of those patients who have not responded to conventional antipsychotic medication. The same series of studies yielded information demonstrating that regular (weekly in most cases) monitoring of blood chemistry, especially in the first six months of treatment, leads to a much lower side effect profile and virtually eliminates the possibility of potentially lethal agranulocytosis.

The apparent success of clozapine led many clinicians to consider broadening its use. However, the prevailing opinion remained that the regular and careful monitoring of blood chemistry required with clozapine limits its usefulness as a first-line treatment. Nevertheless, the research shifted to the development of newer "novel" antipsychotic drugs modeled to varying degrees after clozapine. These newer drugs appear to produce effects similar to those seen with clozapine (improvement of positive symptoms, definite improvement of negative symptoms) relative to conventional treatments, and attain efficacy at doses that do not produce the same degree of extrapyramidal side effects as seen with the conventional treatments. One such drug risperidone is now available world-wide. Other drugs, such as olanzapine, ziprasidone, seroquel and sertindole will soon be available. Together, they constitute a second generation of antipsychotic agents that may be able to treat the entire spectrum of symptoms associated with schizophrenia. And, fortunately, it appears that their effect will be bought at a much smaller cost to the persons suffering from schizophrenia.

As we enter into this new era of drug treatment for schizophrenia, we come face to face with a number of ethical issues. The new generation antipsychotic agents are, at least initially, more expensive than conventional compounds. Their use requires reorientation of practitioners and changes in prescribing habits. Numerous issues remain to be answered regarding their suitability in certain cases and with various types of patients. Yet our overall impression is that they may mark a breakthrough in treatment. This paper confronts these issues in an effort to better understand the dilemma that we will face as more of these medications become available, all promising benefits but with costs that may seem to be too high for overburdened health care systems.

A BIOETHICAL PERSPECTIVE

The ethical issues surrounding the use of conventional antipsychotic medications is best addressed from a bioethical perspective. As we will discuss later in the chapter, the ethics of neuroleptic use embrace such topics as the behaviour of individual physicians, the values of members of the medical and legal communities, the needs of patients, families and caregivers, and the behaviour of the agencies which control or influence health care delivery .

Bioethics provides a broad perspective for the evaluation of patient care issues (Beauchamp and Childress, 1994, Roy, Williams, and Dickens, 1994). It has emerged as a distinct branch of ethics in the last decades of the twentieth century with a distinct goal of providing a well developed and logically consistent framework for discussing the moral/ethical obligations of the health care professionals who work in a rapidly changing, increasingly complex, and technologically driven health care system. At its best, bioethics provides a bridge between traditional ethical theory/moral philosophy, with its broad emphasis on epistemology, and traditional medical ethics with its narrower focus on physician behaviour.

Although there is no single bioethics approach, there are common elements in all treatments of bioethics. These include a commitment to the application of rigorous, analytic techniques to patient-care issues, a focus on topics involving the interface of health care and technology, an attempt to broaden the base of input into ethical issues in health care, and a special concern with the issues of life and death which are faced by health care workers.

Within the traditional medical ethics framework, the standard for ethical behaviour has been shaped by the ancient concept of nonmaleficence (do no harm) and embodied in an approach to practice that sees ethical behaviour in the context of prevailing standards of practice. This has been a justifiable position and has, in fact, ensured that medical practitioners remained true to the prevailing theories and techniques of the time. This approach is consistent with a common sense/common language approach and, in fact, ethics is defined by Webster's Encyclopedic Dictionary as "conforming with an accepted standard of good behavior."

The above definition, however sensible it may seem, does not provide a complete and ethically sound justification (in the broader sense of ethics) for anyones, and particularly a physician's, behaviour. Standards of medical practice change, in response to changes in the medical knowledge base and the development of new therapeutics. As new knowledge and techniques become available, a minority of health care professionals will typically have access to them and will consequently change their patterns of practice. Later, if the changes are widely seen to be positive, the majority of practitioners may follow suit. This creates an interesting situation if one maintains that the final standard of ethical behaviour is conformity with one's colleagues. In fact, the logical result of this interpretation would be the position that cutting edge practitioners are—by definition—acting unethically.

Fortunately, medicine does not actually operate in this way. We recognize that persons operating at the edge of a field may be breaking ground rather than simply creating a mess. Physicians who are operating at the edge often justify their behaviour by reference to other standards than that of common practice -

ypically by demonstrating special expertise or training in an area. But even this oophole does not free one from the adherence to common practice—it merely hifts the focus from generalists to specialists.

Conformity to the behaviour of peers, however, is only one of a number of ways of justifying one's actions. Within bioethics, as within medicine itself, principles other than nonmaleficence are deemed to be valuable. One such principle, and one which is particularly relevant in this instance, is beneficence. Today, we have moved toward a position where physicians are not only enjoined from doing harm, but are equally responsible for promoting good health.

The principle of beneficence has application beyond specific doctor–patient interactions. For example, in the context of general standards of practice, it is now held that while physicians may be bound to follow prevailing standards of practice, they are equally bound to actively work to develop new skills and knowledge that will promote patient care. In the situation of changing medical technology, this means that physicians are bound to work to stay on the edge of developments rather than seeking refuge in the herd. One embodiment of this concern may be seen in the increasingly strong emphasis on continuing medical education. This reflects not only the reality that standards of practice are dynamic rather than static, but that the medical–legal system is expecting a higher standard of behaviour from physicians than has ever been the case. As will be discussed later, the courts are taking a much wider view of physician responsibilities and will not necessarily as an argument that an individual doctor's behaviour is justified simply because other doctors act in the same way.

The question of whether advances in techniques/therapeutics constitute advances in the quality of patient care (the principle of beneficence) is not always easy to determine. This is particularly true when advances involve tradeoffs. For example, a novel therapeutic agent may be more effective, but more expensive, than traditional alternatives. In a world of fixed health care resources, this may necessitate a decision to either increase funding or re-allocate existing program resources. For reasons to be discussed later, the question of resource allocation is particularly problematic when decisions involve mental health funding. Throughout North America there is a demonstrable reluctance to assign psychiatric illness the same priority that we give to such other health care issues as high-risk cardiac surgery, AIDS, and women's health issues. The introduction of these social forces makes the determination of what constitutes ethical behaviour ever more complex.

The bioethical framework provides some assistance in formulating questions that must be answered if one is to make a determination of whether a course of action is defensible. Most health care professional attempt to base decisions on a reasoned analysis of the benefits and costs associated with particular courses of action. The specific techniques that have been introduced to health care decision making to supplement traditional treatment efficacy analyses include classic cost–benefit analysis, cost–effectiveness analyses, risk assessment analyses and so on. The economically focused analyses are seen to be particularly relevant in the case of pharmacological agents used in the treatment of schizophrenia, as many users ultimately depend on some form of government or private insurance funding to pay for their medication. In this case, an ability to reduce costs to the system is often a primary system motivation.

Another type of analysis which is particularly relevant in this context is life quality analysis. For persons with chronic disease, life quality is often a central issue, as failure to achieve a successful treatment response is typically followed by long periods of suffering and incapacitation. Quality of life analysis provides a way of recognizing that increased ability to participate in life, enhanced self-esteem, and the ability to function without institutional supports are tangible benefits. Quality of life analysis allows decision makers to introduce the less objective aspects of treatment into the decision making process. This is particularly important in the analysis of treatment of schizophrenia where life-long incapacitation is still the expected outcome for most people. Sophisticated quality of life analyses are also able to provide at least rough estimates of the economic benefits that accrue to society when people move from being patients to independent, productive members of society.

SETTING THE STAGE

In the previous discussion we have covered several important points. First, the determination of the ethical defensibility of the prescribing habits of physicians is bound to be a complex question. Second, the question of neuroleptics is best seen as a special instance of the general case in which changes in technology set the stage for changes in practice. Third, the question of whether standards should change is best determined from a broad perspective.

If changes in practice can be shown to be beneficial, and if there are demonstrable benefits accruing to the individual and to society, it seems necessary to conclude that change should occur. In the context of this chapter this requires that we must: (1) examine whether the differences between the classes of newer and older drugs are sufficient to determine whether either is more efficacious and beneficial. (2) examine whether the results of exercise one are sufficient to warrant change in prescribing practices. (3) examine whether, in the light of sufficient evidence, the accepted standard has not changed.

Accordingly, we will first look at the literature examining the differences between conventional and novel antipsychotics. Second, we shall examine whether these differences constitute a significant difference such that the prevailing standard of good behaviour. Third, we shall discuss the forces that act to restrict the conditions under which change can occur.

CONVENTIONAL ANTIPSYCHOTICS: EFFICACY

As previously stated, conventional antipsychotics are primarily efficacious in treating the positive or psychotic symptoms of schizophrenia. This is not surprising since they were developed to block the D2 receptor and, consequently, to reverse the psychotic state which has been postulated to be caused by an over-activity of dopamine. Despite being developed specifically to control psychosis, the research indicates that their efficacy is far less than might be expected. In fact, approximately 10–20% of patients show very limited response to D2 agonists and a much large proportion of patients demonstrate partial or incomplete responses to treatment.

The literature on the efficacy of traditional antipsychotics in treating the negative symptoms of schizophrenia is much more equivocal. Review articles (Meltzer et al., 1986; Angst et al., 1989) suggest that they can be effective in treating negative symptoms, but a closer look at this literature suggests that efficacy may not only be dose dependent but that the doses required to achieve therapeutic results are either lower or higher than the dosages normally required for treating psychosis. This in turn suggests that the effect on negative symptoms may occur via different mechanisms than are involved in psychosis. At lower doses there may be a decreased occurrence of drug-induced parkinsonism, likely as a result of the decreased D2 blockade.. A different receptor blockade profile may occur when doses are well above those needed to selectively block the dopamine system. At very high doses, conventional drugs would presumably also block both serotonin and other receptor systems. While this would result in a unique receptor profile, it would no doubt occur at the cost of significant blockade of the dopamine system. This could then be expected to translate into a risk for the development of long-term side effects such as tardive dyskinesia.

This review suggests that conventional antipsychotics have some potential for treating negative symptoms, particularly when used at either low or high dosage levels. Unfortunately, neither strategy can be considered to be optimum. At low dosages, advantages gained in negative symptom response will likely be at a cost of decreased efficacy in treating the psychotic symptoms. Presumably, only that subset of patients who could remain well at lower doses of conventional antipsychotics might show improvement of negative symptoms. When dealing with high-dose strategies, there is also the possibility that long-term exposure to high levels of antipsychotics substantially increases the probability of EPS.

COURSE OF ILLNESS

Until this point, the discussion of efficacy has focused entirely on immediate and short-term improvement. Such a perspective is inherently self-limiting as schizophrenia is a life-long illness. Long-term treatment options are at least as critical as short-term treatments. The impact of conventional antipsychotics on long-term outcome has been examined in a number of studies. Wyatt (1991) suggested that treatment with conventional antipsychotic drugs, in comparison with non-treatment and/or non-drug treatment, improves the long-term course of schizophrenia. This suggests that the natural course of the illness may be altered by intervention with appropriate medication.

The apparent worsening of the disease in the absence of treatment may also indicate a toxicity effect that leads to a general worsening in function following recurring episodes of psychosis. Proponents of this position have not yet fully explicated either the nature of the toxic factor or the mechanism by which this worsening over time might occur. The position, however, is intriguing and argues, together with the empirical data cited above, that treatment of schizophrenia must focus on long-term management. In terms of the issue of whether novel compounds offer a substantial advantage, it is clearly necessary to examine whether novel compounds produce a differentially positive impact on long-term outcome.

CONVENTIONAL ANTIPSYCHOTICS: SIDE EFFECTS

We suggested earlier that efficacy claims are a first line justification for the use of therapeutic agents. The brief review in the previous section demonstrates that efficacy with conventional antipsyhcotics is significant for positive symptoms (although response is less than 100%) and less significant for negative symptoms. Having established that conventional drugs do not fully treat the spectrum of symptoms of schizophrenia, we will now turn to the issue of potential adverse effects of these medications. The presence of adverse effects, particularly if those effects are hazardous to life or well-being, must be considered as a serious problem from both clinical and ethical perspectives. If the principle of nonmaleficence is to be followed, then the use of agents that promote such effects can be justified only if a greater harm might result from not introducing the treatment.

The most serious concern with conventional antipsychotics, it turns out, is not lack of efficacy, or even of limited efficacy. It is the problem of serious side effects. Neuroleptic-induced side effects run the gamut from dry mouth to hormonal alterations and the previously discussed EPS. The prevalence of acute EPS varies widely across studies (Casey, 1991) reflecting perhaps the large number of risk factors including age of the patient, gender, dose of drug and the time course of treatment. Acute EPS are worrisome. Drug-induced parkinsonism, which is similar to idiopathic parkinsonism, can occur and result in dysregulation of motor movements. Patients experiencing this side effect will appear slowed down in their gait and reflexes, and will typically lack facial expression. The secondary effects of EPS include a greater risks for accidents (a result of slowed movements) and a diminished ability to initiate and sustain social interactions (a result of the facial mask phenomenon). The initial decrease in social interaction, in turn, may lead to a longer-term pattern of withdrawal and loss of motivation such that there is an emergence of a syndrome of secondary negative symptoms.

The motor dysregulation that is manifested in tremor and related disorders has a primary effect of reducing people's ability to perform fine motor movements. In addition, disfiguring tremors and other motor disturbances can lead people to avoid social interactions. Just as in the case of slowing and facial masking, this drug-induced change in function can lead to the emergence of a secondary withdrawal from social situations.

Dystonia, a sudden contraction of a muscle or muscle group, is also associated with exposure to traditional antipsychotics. Dystonias can be disfiguring, as in the case of oculgyric crises, painful, as in the case of torticollis, or even life-threatening, as in the case of laryngeal dystonia. Although dystonias may be treated with antiparkinsonian medications, experiencing a dystonia often has a major psychological impact and can lead to a life-long avoidance of treatment.

Finally, akathisia, the subjective experience of intense restlessness, may leave an individual unable to sit still and can eventually both cause difficulties in concentration and result in an exacerbation in any tendency towards violent, even suicidal, behaviour.

In addition to the serious EPS, conventional antipsychotic agents greatly increase the likelihood that a person will develop tardive dyskinesia. Tardive dyskinesia (TD), is an emergent side effect that often results from chronic exposure to conventional antipsychotics. TD is a hyperkinetic syndrome consisting of involuntary abnormal movements of various musculature groups in the body. The term "tardive" is used because this syndrome usually normally develops only after six months or more of conventional therapy. Although TD may be reversible, it is often persistent and irreversible. It can occur in any part of the body and, depending on the location, be either disfiguring, dysfunctional, or both (Yassa and Jones 1985). Disfigurement typically occurs when there are involuntary movement of the facial muscles. Dysfunction can occur when the dyskinesia effects the person's ability to carry out bodily functions. For example dyskinesia of the diaphragm can lead to respiratory irregularities (Wilcox et al. 1995).

The prevalence of TD has been reported to be approximately 15–20% (APA task force Report on Tardive Dyskinesia 1992) for persons treated on a long-term basis with conventional antipsychotic agents. There are also a number of associated tardive abnormalities including tardive dystonia, tardive akathisia, and tardive psychosis. The latter is hypothesized to be a drug-induced tendency to develop psychotic symptoms that is related to compensatory activity in the mesolimbic area (Jones 1995).

SUMMING UP

Returning to our ethics-bound perspective, it seems clear that the side effects issue must be strongly considered in our justification of conventional antipsychotic agents. This opinion is also shared by the public at large and reflected in a number of recent legal decisions. Despite the fact that TD may be an unavoidable result of treatment with conventional antipsychotic agents and that these agents are held to be a first-line treatment of psychosis, the courts have consistently decided in favour of patients with emergent TDs who have sought judgment against the prescribing physician. Clearly the argument that a physician is justified in prescribing *commonly used* therapeutics which produce serious side-effects, *on the basis of an adherence to a common standard of practice*, has been rejected as a first-line defence.

In the context of bioethics, this complex situation raises basic medical practice issues which crystalize around the question of whether the use of conventional antipsychotics, regardless of physician motivation, may in some cases violate the principle of nonmaleficence. This is a moot point as there are data suggesting both positive and negative treatment outcomes. The question of nonmaleficence, in turn, is bound up with an accompanying standard of practice issue, as conventional neuroleptics are indeed the standard therapeutic agent for the vast majority of general and specialist practitioners. To further complicate the issue, the voice of non-medical stakeholders has clearly stated that, regardless of prevailing standards of practice, physicians will be held accountable for the occurrence of serious events in the treatment of their patients—even if they were clearly operating within the nonmaleficence framework.

By moving between ethical, practice, and treatment issues we have come to a higher degree of understanding of the ethical issues of drug use, the clinical features of traditional antipsychotic compounds, and the use of these drugs in practice. We have, in fact, established the following:

Conventional antipsychotics:

1. Are widely used and, by definition, constitute a standard of practice.
2. Are moderately to highly effective in treating psychosis.
3. Are of questionable effectiveness in treating either the primary or secondary negative symptoms of schizophrenia.
4. Have at least a moderate impact on course of illness.
5. Are associated with a wide range of serious side effects.
6. Are perceived by the public and legal experts as dangerous substances that require (a) extreme care in prescribing and (b) acceptance of physician responsibility for the occurrence of side effects.

Fortunately, the discussion does not have to end with these observations. The introduction of new medications has changed the picture and, perhaps, provided a way out of status quo. In the following pages we will argue that the ethical and practice issues may be at least partially resolved by considering the characteristics and treatment roles of atypical neuroleptics.

NOVEL ANTIPSYCHOTICS: EFFICACY

Having already established that conventional antipsychotic agents have limited efficacy and are associated with significant risk of serious side effects, we will now turn to the question of whether novel antipsychotics exhibit comparable or superior efficacy and side-effect profiles to conventional compounds.

POSITIVE SYMPTOMS

We now have considerable evidence that clozapine can be effectively used treat psychotic symptoms in patients who have failed to respond to conventional antipsychotic drug therapies. The literature further suggests that benefits generally become apparent within the first six weeks of treatment and are often maintained through long-term treatment. It remains to be seen whether the benefits documented in the treatment of persons who are non-responsive to conventional therapies will also be seen in a more general patient population. Presently the only data that speaks to this issue was obtained in early studies of the use of acutely psychotic patients. This limited work has suggested that clozapine may show greater efficacy than conventional drug treatments in non refractory patients (Claghorn et al., 1987).

Novel antipsychotic drugs, including risperidone and others that are in development, have not yet demonstrated the same degree of efficacy for psychotic symptoms as has clozapine. Accordingly it is difficult to suggest at thi point that these newer drugs, as a group, have ant general efficacy advantage in treating psychosis over conventional antipsychotics.

In terms of our evaluative framework, the only specific advantage of the novel antipsychotic medications lies in their potential for inducing a response in persons who are non-responsive to conventional medication. The question o differential effects cannot be considered to be fully answered, however, until more controlled studies examining the efficacy of clozapine and other novel medications in treating acute psychosis in a general (non-refractory) population.

NEGATIVE SYMPTOMS.

In the case of negative symptoms, a stronger case can be made for a differential treatment effect between novel and conventional antipsychotics. Whereas with conventional medications, negative symptom response seldom occurs at normal dosages, novel medications may have primary efficacy on negative symptom within the dose range established for treatment of psychosis. Risperidone in particular has demonstrated a differential efficacy in comparison with conventional antipsychotics such as haloperidol (Chouinard et al., 1993) Although the initial reports of this effect were criticized for studying efficacy only against high doses of haloperidol, subsequent studies with other novel antipsychotics have shown that this efficacy is still present at both low fixed doses of haloperidol and when a variable dosing strategy is employed.

Perhaps more importantly, the improvement in negative symptoms does not seem to be related to the emergence of EPS with the comparative medications. As noted earlier, EPS which occur with conventional neuroleptics may produce secondary negative symptoms. The data from comparative studies appear to support a differential treatment effect even in the absence of EPS signs in persons on comparative medications. In other words, the differential response appears to be the result of a primary effect of novel medications rather than a comparison artifact resulting from a higher incidence of EPS in the comparison groups.

Taken as a whole, the available efficacy data suggest that, with respect to positive symptoms, novel antipsychotics demonstrate superior efficacy in treating persons who have proven refractory to conventional medication regimes. With respect to non-refractory patients the data is incomplete but suggestive of efficacy equivalence in treating non-refractory patients. There is also strong evidence that novel antipsychotics possess superior efficacy in treating negative symptoms with the effect attainable at normal dosage levels.

COURSE OF ILLNESS

The next stage of this argument focuses on the impact of novel antipsychotic medication on course of illness. Conventional antipsychotic medications have been shown to have a positive impact on long-term course of illness—at least in comparison with non-drug treatment. Although the mechanism through which such gains are maid is not yet known, the toxicity hypothesis would suggest that the effect is secondary to the control of psychosis. If the toxicity hypothesis is correct, only clozapine, with its well-demonstrated antipsychotic effect, would have a potential advantage over conventional medications. If, however, the effect is related to the ability to prevent relapse, then any drug capable of preventing relapse would, at least theoretically, impact on the course of the disease. There are, in fact, numerous studies suggesting that novel antipsychotics have a differential advantage in preventing relapse (Meltzer and Cola, 1994; Addington et al., 1993). These studies, most of which were promarily concerned with health economic issues, have documented a substantial decrease of relapse and re-admission to hospital in patients treated with novel drugs following earlier exposure to conventional medications.

A question remains as to whether the observed findings are a result of a primary efficacy effect or a simple function of improved compliance with the novel medications—presumably because of the lower side effect profile (see next section). Obviously if a patient continues with medication there may be a better outcome. This does not mean, however, that the medication will not also have an impact on the long-term course of the disorder. Until the proper sequence of studies is carried out, this question will not be fully answered. However, it is reasonable to conclude on the basis of the available data that novel antipsychotics have an advantage in terms of their ability to keep people well over the long term.

NOVEL ANTIPSYCHOTICS: SIDE EFFECTS

The occurrence of serious side effects is a major issue in judging the viability of medications. Although novel antipsychotics such as clozapine have a variety of side effects, the overall profile of novel medications is quite different from that of conventional antipsychotics. The most common side effects with clozapine are an increased risk of seizures and a greater likelihood of blood dyscrasia. Risperidone and other novel medications produce a potent blockade of serotoninergic and adrenergic systems and, in consequence, increase the likelihood of weight gain and possibly sexual dysfunction.

The data that are accumulating for novel medications consistently show that the use of these drugs in standard dosage ranges is not associated with the emergence of EPS. This different profile constitutes a significant advantage. There are two possible explanations of this situation. One is that there is simply a reduced risk of EPS with novel medications. Two, the efficacy of these medications at normal dosages is such that the patient has a greater chance of successful response without requiring dosages high enough to cause significant EPS. This greater chance to be successfully treated without the expected range of side effects is one of the principle means by which novel antipsychotics have distinguished themselves from conventional drugs.

The advantages associated with a reduced side-effect profile are obvious in terms of impact. Avoidance of such side effects such as akathisia, dystonia and parkinsonism, may lead to better function in many aspects of patients' lives. It is also likely that being exposed to a more benign treatment will lead to better compliance rates.

There is a second factor of significance in this situation. If, as has been suggested, emergence of acute EPS predicts later development of chronic EPS such as tardive dyskinesia, then avoidance of acute EPS has significant ramifications for long-term treatment. At the present time it must be considered a hypothesis that novel antipsychotics may be associated with a decreased prevalence of tardive dyskinesia. If, however, the hypothesis is sustainable, then the risk of developing tardive dyskinesia as a result of long-term exposure to antipsychotic drug treatment may be decreased substantially with novel drugs and, in the particular case of clozapine, eliminated.

SUMMING UP

Following the pattern established earlier, we will present the major findings of the review of novel antipsychotic medication. That review established the following points.

Novel antipsychotic agents:

1. Are not yet widely used and, by definition, do not constitute a standard of practice.
2. Are highly effective in treating the psychotic symptoms of persons who have failed to respond to conventional treatment.
3. Have not yet established an advantage in treating acutely ill, non-refractory patients, although the available data suggests that their efficacy is similar to that of conventional medications.
4. Have a proven advantage in treating the negative symptoms of persons with schizophrenia.
5. Have, at the least, a moderate positive impact on relapse, and may also have a primary effect on course of illness.
6. Have a different side effect profile than conventional agents, with significantly lower occurrence of the major side effects of EPS and TD.

In summary, conventional antipsychotic drugs treat primarily the positive or psychotic symptoms of schizophrenia but do not effectively treat the negative symptoms. Their efficacy occurs at doses that induce EPS in a substantial number of patients. Novel antipsychotic drugs do virtually everything that conventional drugs do, with the added advantage of treating secondary negative symptoms better than conventional drugs as well as reducing the occurrence of EPS and TD in the short term and possibly in the long-term as well.

STANDARDS OF PRACTICE

Returning to the bioethical framework established earlier in the chapter, the argument put forward was that if a change in practice could be shown to adhere to the dictum of nonmaleficence and, in addition, that change would result in demonstrable benefits to patients and the public at large, then change should occur. In other words, if primary ethical considerations regarding beneficence and nonmaleficence were to be satisfied then a change in practice should necessarily follow. In terms of our specific case, if the case was established that novel antipsychotic agents are clearly superior to conventional ones in terms of efficacy, side effect profiles, positive effect on course of illness, and ability to lead to improved life quality, it would be reasonable to argue that there is a strong ethics-based argument for a shift in standards of practice.

The previous reviews provide evidence that novel antipsychotic agents are superiors in terms of efficacy, side-effects profiles, effect on course of illness, and ability to improve life quality. With regards to the efficacy information, it is important to recognize that the ability to treat refractory patients confers both a substantial medical advantage and an even greater advantage in terms o improved life quality. Without novel antipsychotic agents, those patients who are refractory to treatment or who are poor responders are condemned to a life without quality, suffering from recurrent, disabling episodes of psychosis and experiencing progressive deterioration and earlier death.

With regard to the later categories of effects, it is worthy of note that the side effect issue has been consistently identified as a critical factor in terms of life quality. As noted in the review of conventional medications, the occurrence o disabling and disfiguring side effects can have devastating consequences for the patient and can lead to both social disablement and a reluctance to participate in medically necessary maintenance treatment. The use of novel agents provides not only an effective treatment alternative but provides hope for a life not only without disabling disease but also with some promise of enhanced life function.

Taken as a whole, the available information points to the clear superiority o novel antipsychotic agents and, within an ethical framework, there are compelling reasons for considering the use of these agents in a much-expanded role. Before making a final pronouncement, however, it is necessary to consider whether, despite the general case for novel agents, there are specific instances in which it would be advantageous and ethically justifiable to use conventional medications.

CIRCUMSTANCES IN WHICH CONVENTIONAL ANTIPSYCHOTICS MAY MAINTAIN AN ADVANTAGE

From a clinical perspective there re several instances in which, despite the previous argument for the primacy of novel antipsychotics, conventional antipsychotic drugs may be considered preferable for the treatment o schizophrenia. The first clear indication for use of conventional drugs would be in the case of patients who require a mode of delivery other than pills. Presently novel antipsychotic drugs are not available in anything other than pill form. If non-compliant patient requires short acting injectable medication then only the conventional drugs that are available in in injectible format can be used Similarly if the patient is unreliable or non-compliant with long term maintenance treatment, it may be only possible to treat effectively with long acting injectable medication. Again, only conventional agents are available in long-acting, injectible format.

The second case is of that of patients who present with predominantly positive symptoms and who might respond to conventional drugs at low doses. This group of patients includes, for example, patients suffering from delusional disorder or positive symptom schizophrenia. These patients may achieve maximum therapeutic benefits when treated with low-dose conventional antipsychotic without experiencing significant side effects. Without disputing the claims for low-dose efficacy, it can be argued that patients exposed to conventional antipsychotics, including those who do not experience acute EPS, remain at risk for development of tardive dyskinesia—particularly if they are maintained on conventional medication for long periods of time. Although the risk would likely be lower with novel antipsychotics, it is difficult to make precise estimates because appropriate studies of low-dose conventional medications in comparison with novel agents have not yet been conducted. Determining whether novel compounds maintain their side-effect advantage against low-dosees conventional medications requires a series of long-term studies.

There is also a clinical/conceptual problem associated with the low dose scenario. It is impossible to predict, except by past history of drug treatment, at which dose patients will begin to show a response to conventional drugs. Consequently clinicians must proceed slowly from dose to dose, hoping that efficacy is achieved before side effects begin to emerge. This procedure both lengthens the time of treatment and increases the risk of these patients developing EPS. And, in fact, if a patient developed acute EPS, the conventional drug therapy would likely be discontinued and the patient switched to novel drug therapy. Unless there is an efficacy advantage for low-dose, conventional antipsychotic agents, the rather cumbersome process which may well end with the prescribing of a novel compound might be avoided.

It appears that there are at least two situations in which the use of conventional medications may be indicated. But it should be noted that in the first case the reason for using conventional antipsychotic agents is purely logistic. The fact that novel antipsychotics are not available in injectible and long-acting format renders the question moot. If it were to be the case, however, that novel medications were available in injectable and long-acting formats, the advantage of conventional medications might well didsappear. In the second case, the justification for using conventional medications is weak. However, until appropriate low-dose comparative studies are carried out, the conventional agents must be presumed to have an advantage with this particular group of patients.

WHEN ARE CONVENTIONAL DRUGS NOT INDICATED

Our final review will focus on a second special issue—those situations other than treatment failures where conventional drugs would not be indicated. Two cases may be identified. The first is that of patients who have responded only partially to conventional drug treatment. The second case is that of patients who are experiencing a first psychotic break. We will examine these special cases keeping in mind that there is not yet a suitable data base to support definitive conclusions.

PARTIAL RESPONDERS

A partial response may include any one, or any combination, of the following:

1. Partial remission of positive symptoms.
2. Persistence of negative symptoms.
3. Emergence of tolerable, although serious, EPS.

Regarding 1, the choice of an alternative treatment would focus first on efficacy and second on side effects. The decision process would focus similar to that in cases of refractory illness. Given the available efficacy data for novel antipsychotics, it is hard to argue that the primary strategy would be to continue with conventional medication. It would seem more reasonable to move to a compound with a better record for producing results with treatment resistant patients. Presently, treatment with clozapine or any other compound with demonstrated strong antipsychotic effect would be justified. One might argue, however, the choice of conventional or novel compounds would be a judgement call focusing on between the balance of efficacy benefits side effect costs.

Regarding 2, the data consistently demonstrates that novel compounds have a decided advantage in treating negative symptoms. Much attention has been given to the clinical problem of distinguishing primary from secondary negative symptoms. Given our knowledge of novel compounds, it seems clear that they bestow a significant advantage, whether it be through the amelioration of secondary negative symptoms or the direct treatment of primary negative symptoms. It is our opinion that it is very hard to justify anything other than a novel medication in this instance.

Regarding 3, the earlier review indicated the number and types of EPS problems—both short and long-term—associated with conventional medications. Even if the EPS experienced by a patient are deemed to be tolerable, the overall situation is unsatisfactory. For one thing, acute EPS may be predictive of later-emerging side effects, notably TD. Given the lower likelihood of this class of side effects occurring with novel medications, it is difficult to justify the use of conventional medications in this situation.

FIRST BREAK PSYCHOSIS

The case of patients who are experiencing a first psychotic episode is more complex. For those patients who have had a prodrome of negative symptoms, novel antipsychotics would be indicated as the drug of first choice. It is conceivable, in this case, that problems could arise if the patient refuses medication in pill form. In such an instance, conventional medications would be indicted until such time as the patient is agreeable to oral medication.

If a patient does not present with negative symptoms it is very difficult to predict whether negative symptoms will eventually arise. From what is known of the natural history of schizophrenia, however, there is a strong likelihood that negative symptoms will become part of the illness. It is also known that emergent EPS following treatment with conventional medications is associated with secondary negative symptoms. In the face of a strong probability that negative symptoms will eventually be part of the illness, the use of novel antipsychotics is also indicated for these patients.

SUMMING UP

A reasonable conclusion seems to be that novel antipsychotic agents are indicated as first-line treatment for patients who are suffering their first break of psychotic illness, for chronically ill patients who are partial treatment responders, and who have either poorly controlled negative symptoms or negative symptoms in conjunction with EPS in the context of conventional drug therapy. The only exception would be those patients who refuse to take their medication by mouth or who cannot reliably manage their medication.

ARE WE CONFORMING WITH A WELL—JUSTIFIED STANDARD?

Returning once again to our ethics-based framework, this final review concludes the analysis of the justification of the use of novel antipsychotic agents. We maintain that the use of novel compounds may be justified in terms if both nonmaleficence and beneficence criteria. If, indeed, novel compounds carry a lower risk factor for either short or long-term side effects and if, as we have argued, the occurrence of side effects is a serious problem, it is impossible to avoid the conclusion that failing to use them (and consequently exposing patients to risk) violates the principle of nonmaleficence. And, given the accumulating data demonstrating the efficacy of novel compounds for treating positive and negative symptoms, there appears to be no seriously competing reason not to use novel agents. The exception would be the special cases described in the last section of the review.

In terms of beneficence criteria, it is also clear that novel compounds carry with them a higher probability of restoring function in difficult to treat patients and a greater likelihood that people will establish and maintain a higher quality of life. The application of life quality techniques to this issue will clearly demonstrate a decided edge for novel compounds over conventional medications. Thus the use of novel compounds is soundly justified in terms of promotion of patients' well-being.

STANDARDS OF PRACTICE ISSUES

If the previous argument is sound, the necessary and next question to be addressed is why medical practice has not already shifted to a widespread use of novel antipsychotic agents. The following section considers some of the reasons for the maintenance of the status quo.

AVAILABILITY

Novel compounds, as their name indicates, are newly developed and not yet available in all jurisdictions. Currently risperidone is the only novel antipsychotic that is available world-wide and without restrictions. Clozapine, the other widely used novel medication, is available only with restrictions and only in some jurisdictions. It is obvious that availability plays a role in use of these medications. However, in many other areas of medicine cutting edge treatment options are no less difficult to access. Nonetheless, they tend to be more heavily used than novel antipsychotics.

The physical availability of novel medications may be one aspect of the access problem. Funding policies often make it difficult for patients to access medications. In Canada, for instance, risperidone usually cannot be used as a first-line treatment unless the patient is able to bear the cost of the medication. While the cost (approximately \$5.00/day) may not seem onerous, most people who need risperidone, or any other novel antipsychotic, are likely to be poor and dependent on government funding for medication. Again, this is an important issue but, in and of itself, does not fully explain the situation. Cost barriers occur with other special treatments for seriously ill people. Our impression, however, is that the barriers are more easily overcome with other populations.

INERTIA

Medicine is generally a conservative profession and there is always a slow start-up in the first months, or sometimes in the first several years, following the introduction of a new treatment. This occurs because it takes time for physicians to learn about the new treatments, to switch patients from conventional treatments and to allow patients to experience the new treatment's benefits. This general slowness of uptake when combined with the inevitable occurrence of treatment failures could account, at least theoretically, for the lag between expert recommendation and change in practice. Such explanations, however, do not appear to account for the overall situation. Risperidone, for example, has now been in use in Canada for approximately three years. During that time there has been extensive education of physicians about this drug. There has also been a considerable amount of expert opinion supporting its use with persons with schizophrenia. Given these parameters it would normally not take three years for an effective treatment to be transitioned.

COST

The third possibility is simply that novel medications cost too much. It is an undeniable fact that the unit costs of risperidone and clozapine are higher than the unit costs of conventional antipsychotics. The product costs, however, are only one aspect of the economic situation and must be balanced against savings that may accrue as a direct result of the use of these medications. This is the essence of cost–benefit analysis. When one takes a cost–benefit perspective, the picture changes. Studies have now demonstrated that decreases in both relapse and rehospitalization, together with a general decrease in mental health service utilization, occur when novel neuroleptics are used (typically clozapine and risperidone). The net result is a substantial saving to the health care system. Evan allowing for the usual lag time in getting clinical information to administrative decision makers, it seems apparent that neither advice from experts nor data from well-designed studies of cost–benefit issues is being acted upon.

As the above commentary suggests, the situation regarding the introduction of novel antipsychotic agents into the health care system is, to say the least, puzzling. There is significant evidence for the efficacy and safety of these drugs. There are compelling reasons to accept the notion that they can lead to improved life quality. There are no compelling economic, availability, or system inertia factors to explain the situation. We are therefore forced to consider that societal values may play a significant role in the overall situation. The discussion will now turn to the question of whether we view mental illness, and schizophrenia in particular, differently than we do other medical disorders.

DO WE ACCEPT A DIFFERENT STANDARD OF TREATMENT FOR SCHIZOPHRENIA?

The question that heads this section may best be answered by considering a second and more general question. If a patient were seriously ill and there was suddenly made available a new treatment that was at least as efficacious as other treatments, was less prone to cause serious side effects, was potentially able to positively alter the course of illness, and had the potential to result in a net cost savings to the health care system, would we deny the patient access to the treatment? The most likely answer for all medically recognized serious illnesses would be an unqualified no.

Having provided an answer to the general question, let us now turn to a specific disorder. If there were two competing treatments of juvenile diabetes, one of which could decrease the secondary consequences of the disorder and could do so without inducing such side effects as hypoglycemia, and could result in a net savings to the system, would we readily accept this treatment. We suggest the answer would be an unqualified yes.

Similarly, if a drug became available that could treat lung cancer even a little better than conventional methods but without inducing the side effects of chemotherapy would we refuse it on the grounds that it cost somewhat more than conventional methods? Although this case is debatable we suspect the answer would be no.

It would be easy to present many more cases in which either society or social policy makers would likely decide that new approaches should be followed, particularly when they have face value. We seem to be predisposed to recognize the value of therapeutic advances and prepared to pay the price for better health care. So why do we drag our feet when the same situation faces us with respect to the treatment of schizophrenia?

It is our contention that the difference between the above examples and the case of novel antipsychotics lies in a general societal tendency to devalue persons with mental illness. Risperidone, for example, costs approximately $5.00 per day at the recommended dosage. This cost is clearly lower than the costs associated with many new (and often less well researched) treatments in other branches of medicine. Yet governments are not willing to fund this treatment. This is truly a puzzling situation. If the data presented in this article are to be believed, $5.00 per day buys a better prognosis for a large number of the seriously ill. The cost for such drugs as AZT is substantially higher and the long-term prognosis poorer, yet governments continue to pay for this and other treatments. One must ask why do these differences exist.

Possibly persons with schizophrenia and their families lack the political clout of better organized interest groups. If this is the case it is a truly unfortunate situation as the abilities of both the patient and the family are diminished—one by the disease itself, the other by the strain of coping with disease—leaving them singularly unable to take on the establishment over funding priorities. We suspect, once again, that this is only part of the picture. The health care system is not yet so amoral as to respond only to special-interest lobbies, although lobbies clearly influence decision making.

Returning for a final time to our ethical framework, we are left with the uneasy conclusion that the treatment of persons with schizophrenia falls far short of the ethical and moral standards of care that we, as a society, seem to maintain for other disadvantaged groups. This conclusion moves us into the area of public ethics and values. While this is too large an issue to fully address fully , but we will offer some thoughts on the matter.

There are many ways to explain this disparity. Sociobiologists and evolutionary psychology, for example, maintain that our social behaviours have been shaped by evolutionary pressures in much the same manner as our physical features (Wright, 1994). Primates, for example, exhibit a tendency to shun members of the group who behave differently, presumably because this restricts mating opportunities and results in certain characteristics being bred out of the gene pool. Humans are hypothesized to have the same predispositions to strangeness. And who better to shun than schizophrenics who are renowned for their strange behaviour. Presumably this reverberates through the system and leads to health care practices that are discriminatory against persons with schizophrenia. There are less elaborate explanations, but they all end at the same point - we engage in discriminatory practices against persons with mental illness.

Tempting as it may seem to explain away our poor treatment of persons with schizophrenia in terms of hardwired genetic predispositions and selected behavioural features, it is just too easy an answer. At some level all behaviour is genetically determined. And at some level all behaviour is environmentally determined. Such superficial analyses ignore the fact that one of the features of being human is the quality of self-reflection and the accompanying ability to change our thoughts and behaviours on the basis of that self-reflective activity. If we accept a lower standard behaviour regarding our treatment of people with mental illness, we also have the ability to recognize that fact and to do something about it. The tolerance of a lower ethical standard for people with mental illness is no more justifiable, on any level, that it would be if the action were directed against a person of a different race, culture, or religion.

The results of our review suggest that a strong ethical case can be made for aggressively pushing for an expanded role for novel antipsychotic agents. The review also suggests that social factors, rather than medical or technological factors stand in the way of achieving a higher standard of care for persons with schizophrenia. Our conclusion is that we have within ourselves and within our society the capacity to change this situation and to move to a higher ethically based standard for the treatment of persons with schizophrenia.

REFERENCES

Addington D.E., Jones B.D., and Bloom D. (1993) Reduction of hospital days in chronic schizophrenic patients treated with risperidone; a respective study.

Angst J., Stassen H.H., and Woggon B. (1989) Effect of neuroleptics on positive and negative symptoms and the deficit state. *Psychopharmacology* 99: S41–S46.

Tardive Dyskinesia: A Task Force Report (1992) (eds. Kane J.M., Jeste D.V., and Barnes T.R.E.), American Psychiatric Association, Washington, DC.

Beauchamp T.L., and Childress J.F. *Principles of Biomedical Ethics* (4th Edition) (1994), Oxford University Press , New York.

Casey D.E.. (1991) Neuroleptic drug–induced extrapyramidal syndromes and tardive dyskinesia. *Schizophrenia Research* 4: 109–120.

Chouinard G., Jones B.D., and Remington G (1993). A Canadian multicentre placebo controlled study of fixed doses of placebo and haloperidol in the treatment of chronic schizophrenic patients. *J. Clin. Pharmacol.*, 13: 25–40.

Claghorn J., Honigfeld G., and Abuzzahab F. (1987) The risks and benefits of clozapine versus chlorpromazine. *J. Clin. Psychopharmacol* 7: 377–384.

Jones B.D. Tardive Psychosis (1995). In *Contemporary Issues in the Treatment of Schizophrenia,* (eds. Shriqui C.L. and Nasrallah H.A.), American Psychiatric Press, Washington , DC.

Kane J.M., Honigfeld G., and Singer J. (1988) Clozapine for the treatment resistant schoizophrenia. *Archives of General Psychiatry* 45: 789–796.

Meltzer H.Y., Sommers A.A., and Luchins D.J. (1996) The effect of neuroleptics and other psychotropic drugs on negative symptoms in schizophrenia. *J. Clin. Psychopharmacol.* 6: 329–338.

Meltzer H.Y., Cola PA (1994) The Pharmacoeconomics of clozapine: a review. *J. Clin. Psych.* 55: Supp.B, 161–165.

Roy, D.J., Williams, J.R., and Dickens, B.M. (1994) Bioethics in Canada. Prentice Hall, Scarborough, Ont.

Talbott, J.A. (1994) Lessons Learned About the Chronic Mentally Ill Since 1955. In *Schizophrenia: Exploring the Spectrum of Psychosis* (eds. Ancill, R.J., Holliday, S., and Higenbottam J.), John Wiley & Sons, Chichester.

Wilcox P.G., Bassett A., Jones B.D., and Fleetham J.A. (1994): Respiratory dysrhythmias in patients with tardive dyskinesia. *Chest 105:* 203–207.

Wright R. (1994) The Moral Animal. Vintage Books, New York.

Wyatt R.J. (1991) Neuroleptics and the natural course of schizophrenia. *Schizophrenia Bull.* 17: 235–280.

Yassa R. and Jones B.D. (1985) Complications of tardive dyskinesia: a review. *Psychosomatics* 26: 305–313

8

HIGH DOSE ANTIPSYCHOTICS: RISK/BENEFIT CONSIDERATION

Malcolm Lader

In 1980, Aubrée and I reviewed the use of high and ultra-high dose antipsychotic medication and concluded that "high doses of neuroleptics are at least as effective as standard dosage" but that "unwanted effects, especially of the extrapyramidal type, are more severe and frequent." And: "high dose regimens should only be resorted to after dosages given for an adequate trial have been unsuccessful." Since that time, new and atypical antipsychotic drugs have been introduced, the most notable being clozapine. Other interesting compounds are under development. The risk/benefit ratios of these drugs vary greatly. Thus, clozapine is perceived as highly effective but carrying a major risk of blood dyscrasia: typically it is licensed for the treatment of otherwise treatment-resistant patients. By contrast, risperidone is perceived as having a low risk of side effects, at least in moderate dosage, and of being effective in many patients. Its efficacy in treatment-resistant patients is still under investigation.

Growing awareness of serious adverse effects such as the neuroleptic malignant syndrome and reports of sudden death have led to a re-evaluation of the risks of antipsychotic medication. For example, the Royal College of Psychiatrists issued detailed guidelines but for how to rather than whether to use high dose regimens (Thompson, 1994). It seems appropriate, therefore, to review as critically as possible the risks and benefits of high dose medication in the management of psychotic patients both in hospital and in the community.

Schizophrenia: Breaking Down the Barriers. Edited by S.G. Holliday, R.J. Ancill and G.W. MacEwan. © 1996 John Wiley & Sons Ltd.

The theme of this conference is "Breaking down the barriers." There is little point in doing so if the patient "freed" from the restraints of hospital incarceration is then shackled by the ineffectiveness of his/her treatment or the side effects of antipsychotic medication. Should high doses ever be used and if so, are they safe?

WHAT IS A HIGH DOSE?

The general definition of a high dose is one where the "total daily dose exceeds the advisory upper limit for general use." This is generally taken to be the level stated in the Data Sheet or in the relevant National Formulary (see Table 1).

Table 1. Advisory Maximum Daily Oral Doses from the British National Formulary.

Drug	Dose: mg
Chlorpromazine	1000
Clozapine	900
Droperidol	120
Haloperidol	100
	(occasionally 200)
Loxapine	250
Pimozide	20
Remoxipride	600
Risperidone	16
Sulpiride	2400
Thioridazine	800

Having been myself involved in the past in helping to draw up Data Sheets and in advising the British National Formulary, this definition really begs the question. Very often the upper limit is vague, or is non-existent, or is based on usage rather than a careful evaluation of the risk/benefit ratio at various dosage levels. Furthermore, dosage ranges will depend on other factors such as age, bodyweight, use of other medication and so on. What is clear, however, is that the total antipsychotic load is what matters. Polypharmacy with several drugs each at recommended maximum limits does not constitute safe prescribing.

The problem is best turned on its head. Usual therapeutic ranges can be defined from the efficacy data relating to each drug, particularly those introduced more recently. Then, by definition, any dose which exceeds the upper limit for which adequate controlled data are available is "high dose."

THE EFFECTS OF ANTIPSYCHOTICS

Much of our perception of the indications for antipsychotic medication, particularly in conservative prescribing nations like the UK, stems from the properties of the prototypal compound, chlorpromazine. This drug was developed in the search for a better antihistamine. It has strong central antihistaminic actions and is consequently quite sedating as well as having antipsychotic effects. Others, such as haloperidol, are much less sedating.

Let us describe more carefully what we mean. Antipsychotic actions reduce or eliminate the intensity of psychotic phenomena such as delusions, hallucinations, feelings of passivity, thought disorder and inappropriate mood. Typically, the effect is delayed, suggesting (as with the antidepressants) that some secondary process is associated with the therapeutic response and not just prompt dopamine blockade. Many of the unwanted effects, particularly the extrapyramidal ones, are linked to the dopamine blockade, and some, such as dystonias, are rapid in onset. The sedative actions are much less specific and relate to other pharmacological properties, mainly antihistaminic and perhaps antiadrenergic. This is an immediate effect in most cases but closely resembles the sedative actions of other agents such as the benzodiazepines and the older compounds such as the barbiturates and paraldehyde.

There is possibly yet a third action. The efficacy of antipsychotic medication is not closely related to dopamine receptor occupancy (Farde et al., 1992). Thus, modest doses of chlorpromazine and thioridazine (300–400 mg/day), haloperidol and pimozide (4–12 mg/day) and flupenthixol (6 mg/day) occupy 70–90% of dopamine receptors, as visualised by PET or SPECT, and appropriate ligands. Furthermore, risperidone occupies both dopamine-2 and 5-HT$_2$ receptors at quite low doses (Nyberg et al., 1993). Clozapine has enhanced efficacy, yet is a weak antagonist of D$_2$ receptors, and has many other actions, the relevance of which to its efficacy profile remains unclear (Wagstaff and Bryson, 1995). For all these reasons, we should be cautious in ascribing antipsychotic action to direct dopamine blockade (Mackay, 1994). Unfortunately, our ignorance of the precise mode of action of antipsychotic drugs precludes any rational analysis of the dose–response relationships, necessitating reliance on the empirical establishment of risks and benefits at various doses.

HOW ARE ANTIPSYCHOTIC DRUGS USED?

Although three or even four broad treatment situations are generally envisaged, the boundaries between them are indistinct and sometimes therapeutic goals are multiple. For example, an acutely disturbed psychotic patient may need immediate calming but it is hoped that the medication will also help to lessen the psychotic features of the illness, but perhaps on a somewhat longer time scale.

A. EMERGENCY TREATMENT

Psychotic patients are often violent and aggressive (Wistedt and Palmstierna, 1991). This can be a problem even in a closed psychiatric ward (Omerov et al., 1991) where the staff are trained to deal with such incidents and medical help is on hand. In the community, such occurrences are uncommon but come readily to public notice and may be magnified by media interest. Furthermore, the public-at-large is rightly wary of the aggressive mentally ill and the forces of law-and-order, the police for example, may overreact. In one incident in my medico-legal practice, eight police in full riot gear were mobilised to deal with one patient—admittedly rather a large one!

Whatever the circumstances, recourse is usually made to medication, typically parenteral antipsychotics. In the UK, chlorpromazine or haloperidol, or more recently droperidol, are the favourites for such "rapid tranquillisation" (Pilowsky et al., 1992). However, a recent survey (Simpson and Anderson, 1996) of 69 senior and junior psychiatrists showed practice to vary widely. Two unsatisfactory therapies were cited. Thus 22% of respondents stated that they would use intramuscular diazepam, despite ample evidence in the literature that absorption of diazepam by this route is erratic, delayed and unpredictable. (This contrasts with i.m. lorazepam which is rapidly effective.) Even worse, half the respondents would use a depot antipsychotic for rapid tranquillisation despite the total irrationality of this manoeuvre!

Increasing use is being made of benzodiazepines in emergency situations. This is to be commended as they are effective tranquillisers and fairly safe, even in high doses (Glod, 1994). Furthermore, any toxic effects such as respiratory depression can be reversed by the specific benzodiazepine antagonist, flumazenil. There are no specific antidotes to the antipsychotic drugs. Unfortunately, very few controlled studies have evaluated various medications in emergency situations (Dubin, 1988), and a more systematic probing of the whole problem is required. The cost of containing violent and aggressive patients in psychiatric intensive care units (PICUs) is quite substantial so that reduction in the need for such care by judicious use of medication would result in useful cost savings (Hyde and Harrower-Wilson, 1995).

B. ACUTE TREATMENT

The vogue for "rapid neuroleptization" seems to have lessened. In this technique, high doses of antipsychotic drugs (neuroleptics) are given in the first few weeks of hospitalization in order to accelerate the remission of psychotic symptoms (Table 2). Studies of this approach, however, showed it to be no more effective than standard or conservative dosage schedules (e.g. Neborsky et al., 1981; Donlon et al., 1980; Coffman et al., 1987; Rifkin et al., 1991).

Table 2. Symptoms of Schizophrenia

Symptoms:	
Thought disorder	- blocking, deprivation, insertion
	- primary delusions—persecution
	- grandeur
	- hypochondriacal
Sense deceptions	- hallucinatory voices
	heat, cold
	pain, shock
Emotional disorders	- flattening
	- incongruity
Behavioural disturbances	- passivity, destructiveness, aggression and hostility.
	- catatonic stupor
	- negativism, mannerisms

Nevertheless, it is common and legitimate practice to use medium-to-high doses during the early phases of an acute relapse. Unfortunately, these doses are often maintained too long with the emergence of troublesome side effects such as akathisia or over-sedation. In the UK, clopixol acuphase is often favoured. It is a longer-acting drug, given by i.m. injection, and lasting up to 72 hours.

C. MAINTENANCE THERAPY

As with antidepressants, current practice with antipsychotic medication is tending more and more to involve long-term or even life-long maintenance treatment. The time-frame of relapse occurs along an exponential function suggesting that the number of patients relapsing remains a constant proportion of those remaining at risk (Davis, 1975; Davis et al., 1980). Most, perhaps almost all, of patients with an established diagnosis of schizophrenic psychosis will eventually relapse unless maintained on antipsychotic medication. Even after years of stabilization on such medication with no relapses, patients will run the risk of relapse if switched over to placebo.

Long-term medication is fraught with problems both of emergent unwanted effects such as tardive dyskinesia and failure to comply adequately with medication (Weiden et al., 1991). The issue of non-compliance is generally addressed by the use of depot antipsychotics (Davis et al., 1994). The rate of non-compliance drops from about 30% to about 10% and of course becomes overt if the patient fails to come for treatment. Nevertheless, some patients fail to respond even to high doses of depot medication. The non-compliant ones are often the more ill, the non-compliance both resulting in relapse and acting as a marker for incipient relapse. Hence the great debate about compulsory treatment in the community, a dispute which fails to recognize the limitations of antipsychotic therapy.

Later in the illness, negative symptoms of withdrawal and poor motivation may come to dominate the clinical picture. Some negative symptoms are secondary to positive symptoms, for example, social isolation as a consequence of paranoid delusions. Others are primary, have often been present throughout the illness and have been masked by the positive symptoms. Many of these negative features antedate the onset of the acute illness. By and large, treating primary negative symptoms with drugs is an unrewarding experience.

D. THE TREATMENT-RESISTANT PATIENT

In each of the above situations, at least 10% and sometimes closer to 30% of patients fail to respond adequately to drug treatment. The acutely disturbed behaviour may be slow to subside, or the acute episode show few signs of abating, or the chronic patient continues to have florid and/or handicapping symptoms (Table 3). Very often the dosages are pushed up until side effects preclude any further increase or partial response is seen. The problem of such patients has been thrown into sharper relief by the advent of clozapine (Wagstaff and Bryson, 1995).

Table 3. Treatment Resistance in Schizophrenic Patients

Treatment - resistant:
(about 25% of patients)

No response during acute phase

Inexorable downward course

Repeated relapse

Residual symptoms - positive
                            - negative
Chronic deficit state

Refractory depression

Clozapine was originally developed in the 1960s and was regarded favourably until the occurrence of fatal agranulocytosis in Finland in 1975. Development of clozapine was suspended but it remained prescribable in some countries such as Germany. Eventually it was shown to have unique efficacy in schizophrenia and to have an acceptably low incidence of blood dyscrasias with careful blood monitoring (Kane, 1993). However, its indication is generally for treatment-resistant schizophrenic patients or those intolerant of standard medications (Farmer and Blewett, 1993). Its advocates urge its wider usage (e.g. Kerwin, 1996), but others remain lukewarm as to its merits even now (e.g. Jalenques, 1996).

As mentioned earlier, the mode of action of clozapine remains unresolved (Kerwin, 1994). It is a "dirty" drug, binding to a plethora of receptors. However, study of its pharmacology has spawned a series of hypotheses, and modern pharmaceutical chemistry has the means to synthesise molecules to put the various hypotheses to the test (Pickar, 1995).

THE USE OF HIGH DOSES

Debate continues as to whether the use of high doses is ever justified. A consensus has emerged that high doses are not indicated as an initial treatment, but it remains an open issue as to whether they are justified if normal doses have failed (Hirsch and Barnes, 1994). Why is this?

The answer lies in the paucity, perhaps absence, of data from studies designed specifically to address this issue. Comparison of normal and high doses answers a different question. What is needed are studies in which patients who have failed to respond to normal doses of medication are allocated randomly and double-blind to either continue on the same dose or be treated with a higher dose. Otherwise, improvement on a higher dose after failure to respond to a lower dose may merely reflect the passage of time and spontaneous remission.

Despite this lacuna of evidence-based practice, some patients do attain high doses of medication and appear to relapse if the dosage is lowered. From the bulk of such clinical anecdotal evidence, it would seem that high doses can be justified on efficacy grounds in some patients. What proportion of all patients this represents is unclear. Because these patients on high doses develop complications they tend to be more apparent to the clinician who probably overestimates their frequency. This is particularly evident when psychiatric care is shared between primary and secondary care, the treatment-refractory and side-effect-sensitive patients tending to gravitate to the specialist. Forensic patients also tend to be disproportionately in the limelight, and to be treated with high doses, although the advent of clozapine is capable of lessening this problem (Buckley et al., 1995).

UNWANTED EFFECTS

The other half of the equation concerns unwanted effects (Table 4). Most are dose-related, a notable exception being agranulocytosis with clozapine (Mendelowitz et al. 1995). The unwanted side-effects of antipsychotic drugs have been reviewed exhaustively (e.g. Schwartz and Brotman, 1992; Edwards and Barnes, 1993), often concentrating on the extrapyramidal effects, particularly on long-term use (Bristow and Hirsch, 1993; Cavallaro and Smeraldi, 1995; Sachdev, 1995). I shall confine myself to three topics of particular interest to me, stemming from both my clinical and medico-legal experience.

Table 4. Relative Potency and Tolerability of Antipsychotic Agents (from Schwartz and Brotman, 1992, with permission)

Drug	Approximate equivalent (mg)	Relative potency[b]	Adverse effects			
			Anticholinergic effects	sedation	hypotension	extra-pyramidal effects
Phenothiazines						
Aliphatic						
Chlorpromazine	100	Low	+ + + +	+ + + + +	+ + + + +	+ +
Piperadines						
Mesoridazine	50	Low	+ + +	+ + +	+ + +	+ +
Thioridazine	90 - 100	Low	+ + + + +	+ + + +	+ + + + +	+
Piperazinees						
Fluphenazine	2	High	+ +	+ +	+ +	+ + + + +
Perphenazine	10	Intermediate	+ +	+ +	+ +	+ + +
Trifluoperazine	5	High	+ +	+	+ +	+ + + +
Thioxanthenes						
Chlorprothixene	100	Low	+ + + +	+ + + +	+ + + +	+ + +
Thiothixene	3 - 5	High	+ +	+ +	+ +	+ + + +
Dibenzapines						
Clozapine	150	Low	+ + +	+ + +	+ + +	
Loxapine	10 - 15	Intermediate	+ + +	+ + +	+ +	+ + +
Indoles						
Molindole	8 - 10	Intermediate	+++	+	+ +	+ + +
Butryophenones						
Haloperidol	2 - 3	High	+	+ +	+	+ + + + + +
Diphenylbutylpiperidines						
Pimozide	2 - 3	High		+ +	+	+ + + + +

a Dose equivalent to chlorpromazine 100 mg
b Relative affinity for D_2 postsynaptic receptors

A. SUDDEN DEATH

Disquiet has been expressed for many years over the possibility that antipsychotic drugs, particularly in high doses, are associated with an increased risk of sudden death (Table 5). The most authoritative statement on the matter, reviewing the data up to the mid-1980's, concluded as follows (Task Force Report, 1987): "Although a relationship between the use of antipsychotic drugs and sudden death has not been firmly established, it also has not been disproven. From a neurocardiologic perspective, these drugs have the potential for both increasing and decreasing the risk of sudden death. Ultimate outcome is probably determined by a multitude of interacting factors, and the role played by the drug in a given individual is difficult, if not impossible, to determine." Has anything changed to help us firm up this vague and rather unhelpful, fence-sitting conclusion?

Table 5. Mechanisms of Death in Psychiatric Patients

Hypotension
Post-ictal
Aspiration
Megacolon
Heat stroke
Neuroleptic malignant syndrome
Physical exhaustion - mania
       - lethal catatonia
Stress factors

Firstly, 24-hour ambulatory EKG recordings now reveal fairly frequent cardiac abnormalities even in ostensibly normal subjects. For example, in one series of 156 recordings, only 20 (13%) showed normal sinus rhythm throughout (Stinson et al., 1995). The commonest abnormality was supraventricular ectopics and unsustained ventricular tachycardia was seen in three recordings. It would appear, therefore, that a small proportion of even young normal subjects have cardiac rhythm abnormalities of clinical importance, and of particular relevance when drugs with actions on the heart are administered.

Secondly, sudden death in apparently normal subjects is by no means rare, especially in situations of exertion as in sport (Hillis et al., 1994). The parallels to the struggling psychiatric patient are apparent. Cardiac pathology may be present: in the younger patient, hypertrophic cardiomyopathy may be a particular risk.

n a preliminary paper, Jusic and I outlined eight medico-legal cases in which
blood samples had been taken after sudden unexpected death, and analysed for
drug concentrations (Jusic and Lader, 1994). Of these eight, five patients had
high or very high concentrations of antipsychotic and/or an antidepressant drug.
Even taking into account the problems of interpreting post-mortem drug
concentrations (Pounder and Jones, 1990), the reasonable conclusion is that high
bodily concentrations of antipsychotic drugs carry an increased risk of sudden
death. Since publication of this paper, my medico-legal series of sudden deaths
in psychiatric patients has increased to about 30. At least two-thirds seem to be
cardiac in mechanism, the others being respiratory, or following embolism or
epileptic fits. The following factors seem germane:

1. Pre-existing cardiac pathology such as coronary stenosis, myocardial
   hypertrophy, or a conduction defect such as a "long QT syndrome."
2. A struggling patient—this releases adrenaline which sensitises the heart.
3. High drug concentrations, reflecting either high doses, extremely slow
   metabolism or a drug interaction, often between an antipsychotic and an
   antidepressant drug.
4. Respiratory depression—due to medication or an infection—which causes
   anoxaemia of the heart muscle.

It is uncertain how frequent this occurrence is. A survey in Finland (population
.25 million) revealed 49 cases in three years (Mehtonen et al., 1991). This
works out as three or so per million per year. Extrapolating to the UK (adult
population about 56 million), this is over 150 cases/year, that is one every two
weeks or so. My own experience accords with this high rate. Currently, surveys
are being carried out to establish the incidence of this tragic occurrence.

NEUROLEPTIC MALIGNANT SYNDROME (NMS)

This is a puzzling syndrome which still generates much controversy (Bristow
and Kohen, 1993). It is described as having four classical signs—hyperthermia,
rigidity, autonomic dysfunction and altered consciousness. Many dispute that it
is a distinct syndrome but regard it as an extreme example of an extrapyramidal
disorder (Gratz and Simpson, 1994).

A review of 115 cases uncovered 107 cases in which it was known which
antipsychotic drug was being administered at the time the NMS supervened
(Addonizio et al., 1987). High-potency antipsychotic drugs such as haloperidol
were particularly frequently mentioned but this may reflect usage rather than a
specific association. Also, depot antipsychotic medication was often involved.

The relationship of dosage to the development of NMS is controversial. It is generally accepted as a risk factor (e.g. Keck et al., 1989), but rate of increase of dosage rather than the actual dosage itself may be more important. Combinations of antipsychotic drugs, or combinations with other drugs such as lithium or an antidepressant, may constitute a special risk. Again, this may result in antipsychotic drug concentrations higher than those intended. Reintroduction of the offending antipsychotic drug is usually safe, providing a drug-free interval of two weeks is left, and dosages are modest. This militates against NMS being a hypersensitivity phenomenon.

Although the features are fairly characteristic, I have encountered several cases where the diagnosis was by no means clear. Alternative diagnoses include catatonic stupor, malignant hyperthermia, heat stroke and, with combination therapy, lithium toxicity.

The incidence is around 1% which is quite high considering the number of patients taking antipsychotic medication. It is my impression that milder forms of NMS go unrecognized, being dismissed as a hyperthermic spike in a patient with marked extrapyramidal signs. Estimation of creatine kinase is often misleading rather than helpful: many patients with elevated kinase levels are not suffering from NMS. Withdrawal of medication may then precipitate a relapse in the psychotic illness.

IMPAIRMENT OF COGNITIVE FUNCTION

I first became interested in this adverse effect when I was a subject in a study of chlorpromazine and noted marked impairment of psychomotor and cognitive function. I felt "like a zombie" as patients often describe the experience. However, the literature is by no means consistent (King, 1990), psychological impairment not being a routine finding with antipsychotic medication in patients. Why is this?

Schizophrenic patients are themselves functioning psychologically at a reduced level. A recent study tested 36 treatment-refractory schizophrenic patients before the initiation of clozapine therapy (Hagger at al., 1993). Compared with 26 normal controls, the patients, largely drug-free, were impaired with respect to memory, attention and executive function. These impairments were not marginal but averaged a 30% drop in functioning.

With antipsychotic drug therapy in unselected psychotic patients, two processes ensue. The majority, say 70%, of patients improve in their mental state and this is accompanied by an improvement in psychological functioning. However, the antipsychotic drug therapy, itself, may have a sedating effect and this is associated with an impairment in functioning (Cassens et al., 1990). This impairment is strongly dose-related. The net result will depend on the relative strengths of the two effects so that patients may be impaired, improved or roughly the same (King, 1990). The patients who are most disadvantaged are those who fail to respond therapeutically but who develop marked sedation as a side effect.

Two factors can mitigate the impairment. Firstly, if a good therapeutic response eventuates, this will outweigh the direct sedation-related impairment. This happened in the Hagger et al. (1993) study where clozapine improved performance despite its marked sedative effects because patients improved in their psychopathology. Secondly, because the sedative effect of antipsychotic medication is strongly dose-related, conservative dosage regimens will lessen the "load" on the patient, and should lessen "negative" views of medication (Windgassen, 1992).

CONCLUSIONS

Schizophrenia is a severe and indeed life-shortening disorder. A review of the literature shows a mortality ratio of around twice normal (Allebeck, 1989). It is not surprising that strenuous efforts are made by many psychiatrists and their care teams to control the symptoms and prevent relapse. Nevertheless, up to 30% of patients show an inadequate response and it is understandable that higher and higher doses are resorted to in desperate attempts to help the patient, family and carers.

It is my contention that high dose therapy has been shown not to be associated with a better outcome than normal doses. To give further authority for this: a meta-analysis by Bollini and her colleagues (1994) of 22 randomized controlled trials found no therapeutic advantage in using doses above 375 mg/day equivalent of chlorpromazine, whereas adverse effects increased significantly in frequency. Thus, routine use of high doses cannot be sanctioned on the basis of controlled evidence. If in an individual case the clinician decides to escalate the dose, he should do so with care, keeping an open mind, and continuously monitoring the risk/benefit ratio against the severity of the condition.

Too often, therapeutic vigour and optimism have outrun safety considerations. Both common side effects such as sedation and uncommon, but not rare ones, such as NMS and sudden death must be firmly entered as part of the therapeutic equation. The outcome in schizophrenia is poor, less than half of sufferers having a satisfactory long-term outcome. And, unfortunately, this outcome has not materially improved with the advent of antipsychotic medication (Hegarty, 1994). The use of such medication must be just one element in a wide-ranging management plan (see Table 6).

Table 6. Management of Schizophrenia

Management:

- psychological
- family (heavy burden)
- social
- hospital admission
- behavioural, e.g. "token economies"
- drug - dopamine - blocking agents - chlorpromazine, haloperidol,
  depot injections & etc.

REFERENCES

Addonizio G., Susman V.L., and Roth S.D. (1987) "Neuroleptic malignant syndrome: review and analysis of 115 cases", *Biol Psychiatry*, 22, 1004–1020.

Allebeck P. (1989) "Schizophrenia: a life–shortening disease", *Schizophr Bull*, 15, 81–89.

Aubrée J.C., and Lader M.H. (1980) "High and very high dosage antipsychotics: a critical review", *J Clin Psychiatry*, 41, 341–350.

Bollini P., Pampallona S., Orza M.J., Adams M.E., and Chalmers T.C. (1994) "Antipsychotic drugs: is more worse? A meta–analysis of the published randomized control trials", *Psychol Med*, 24, 307–316.

Bristow M.F., and Hirsch S.R. (1993) "Pitfalls and problems of the long term use of neuroleptic drugs in schizophrenia", *Drug Safety*, 8, 136–148.

Bristow M.F., and Kohen D. (1993) "How 'malignant' is the neuroleptic malignant syndrome?", *Br Med J*, 307, 1223–1224.

Buckley P.F., Kausch O., and Gardner G. (1995) "Clozapine treatment of schizophrenia: implications for forensic psychiatry", *J Clin Forensic Med*, 2, 9–16.

Cassens G., Inglis A.K., Applebaum P.S., and Gutheil, T.G. (1990) "Neuroleptics: effects on neuropsychological function in chronic schizophrenic patients", *Schizophr Bull*, 16, 477–499.

Cavallaro R., and Smeraldi E. (1995) "Antipsychotic–induced tardive dyskinesia. Recognition, prevention and management", *CNS Drugs*, 4, 278–293.

Coffman J.A., Nasrallah H.A., Lyskowski J. et al. (1987) "Clinical effectiveness of oral and parenteral rapid neuroleptization", *J Clin Psychiatry*, 48, 20–24.

Davis J.M. (1975) "Overview: maintenance therapy in psychiatry. 1: Schizophrenia", *Am J Psychiatry*, 132, 1237–1245.

Davis J.M., Dysken M.W., Haberman S.J. et al. (1980) "Use of survival curves in analysis of antipsychotic relapse studies", *Adv Biochem Psychopharmacol*, 24, 471–481.

Davis J.M., Metalon L., Watanabe M.D., and Blake L. (1994). "Depot antipsychotic drugs. Place in therapy", *Drugs*, 47, 741–773.

Dubin W.R. (1988) "Rapid tranquilization: antipsychotics or benzodiazepines?", *J Clin Psychiatry*, 49 (Suppl.12), 5–11.

Donlon P.T., Hopkin J.T., Tupin J.P., et al. (1980). "Haloperidol for acute schizophrenic patients: an evaluation of three oral regimens", *Arch Gen Psychiatry*, 37, 691–695.

Edwards J.G., and Barnes T.R.E. (1993) "The side–effects of antipsychotic drugs. II. Effects on other physiological systems.", *Antipsychotic Drugs and their Side–effects* (Ed. T.R.E. Barnes), Academic Press, London.

Farde L., Nordstrom A.L., Wiesel F.A. et al. (1992) "Positron emission tomographic analysis of central D1 and D2 dopamine receptor occupancy in patients treated with classical neuroleptics and clozapine", *Arch Gen Psychiatry*, 49, 538–544.

Farmer A.E., and Blewett A. (1993) "Drug treatment of resistant schizophrenia. Limitations and recommendations", *Drugs*, 45, 374–383.

Glod C.A. (1994) "Major uses of psychopharmacology in the emergency department", *J Emerg Nurs*, 20, 33–40.

Gratz S.S., and Simpson G.M. (1994) "Neuroleptic malignant syndrome. Diagnosis, epidemiology and treatment", *CNS Drugs*, 2, 429–439.

Hagger C., Buckley P., Kenny J.T., Friedman L., Ubogy D., and Meltzer H.Y. (1993). "Improvement in cognitive functions and psychiatric symptoms in treatment–refractory schizophrenic patients receiving clozapine", *Biol Psychiatry*, 34, 702–712.

Hegarty J.D., Baldessarini R.J., Tohen M., Waternaux C., and Oepen G. (1994). "One hundred years of schizophrenia: a meta–analysis of the outcome literature", *Am J Psychiatry*, 151, 1409–1416.

Hillis W.S., McIntyre P.D., Maclean J., Goodwin J.F., and McKenna W.H. (1994). "Sudden death in sport", *Br Med J*, 309, 657–660.

Hirsch S.R., and Barnes T.R.E. (1994). "Clinical use of high–dose neuroleptics", *Br J Psychiatry*, 164, 94–96.

Hyde C.E., and Harrower–Wilson C. (1995). "Resource consumption in psychiatic intensive care: the cost of aggression", *Psychiatr Bull*, 19, 73–76.

Jalenques I. (1996). "Drug–resistant schizophrenia. Treatment options", *CNS Drugs*, 5, 8–23.

Jusic N., and Lader M. (1994). "Post–mortem antipsychotic drug concentrations and unexplained deaths", *Br J Psychiatry*, 165, 787–791.

Kane J.M. (1993). "Newer antipsychotic drugs. A review of their pharmacology and therapeutic potential", *Drugs*, 46, 585–593.

Keck Jr. P.E., Pope Jr. H.G., Cohen B.M. et al. (1989). "Risk factors for neuroleptic malignant syndrome. A case–control study", *Arch Gen Psychiatry*, 46, 914–918.

Kerwin R.W. (1994). "The new atypical antipsychotics. A lack of extrapyramidal side–effects and new routes in schizophrenia research", *Br J Psychiatry*, 164, 141–148.

Kerwin R.W. (1996). "An essay on the use of new antipsychotics", *Psychiatr Bull*, 20, 23–29.

King D.J. (1990). "The effect of neuroleptics on cognitive and psychomotor function", *Br J Psychiatry*, 157, 799–811.

Mackay A.V.P. (1994). "High–dose antipsychotic medication", *Adv Psychiatr Treatment*, 1, 16–23.

Mehtonen O–P., Aranko K., Mälkonen L., and Vapaatalo H. (1991). "A survey of sudden death associated with the use of antipsychotic or antidepressant drugs: 49 cases in Finland", *Acta Psychiatr Scand*, 84, 58–64.

Mendelowitz A.J., Gerson S.L., Alvir J. Ma J., and Lieberman J.A. (1995). "Clozapine–induced agranulocytosis. Risk factors, monitoring and management", *CNS Drugs*, 4, 412–421.

Neborsky R., Janowsky D., Munson E. et al. (1981). "Rapid treatment of acute psychotic symptoms with high– and low–dose haloperidol", *Arch Gen Psychiatry*, 38, 195–199.

Nybert S., Farde L., Eriksson L., Halldin C., and Eriksson B. (1993). "5–HT$_2$ and D$_2$ dopamine receptor occupancy in the living human brain", *Psychopharmacology*, 110, 265–272.

Omerov M., Wistedt B., and Durling U. (1991). "Aggressive incidents in psychiatric wards", *Nord J Psychiatry*, 45 (Suppl. 25), 13–16.

Pickar D. (1995). "Prospects for pharmacotherapy of schizophrenia", *Lancet*, 345, 557–562.

Pilowsky L.S., Ring H., Shine P.J., Battersby M., and Lader M. (1992). "Rapid tranquillisation. A survey of emergency prescribing in a general psychiatric hospital", *Br J Psychiatry*, 160, 831–835.

Pounder D.J., and Jones G.R. (1990). "Post–mortem drug redistribution—a toxicological nightmare", *Forensic Science International*, 45, 253–263.

Rifkin A., Doddi S., Karajgi B. et al. (1991). "Dosage of haloperidol for schizophrenia", *Arch Gen Psychiatry*, 48, 166–170.

Sachdev P. (1995). "The identification and management of drug–induced akathisia", *CNS Drugs*, 4, 28–46.

Schwartz J.T., and Brotman A.W. (1992). "A clinical guide to antipsychotic drugs", *Drugs*, 44, 981–992.

Simpson D., and Anderson I. (1996). "Rapid tranquillisation: a questionnaire survey of practice", *Psychiatr Bull*, 20, 149–152.

Stinson J.C., Pears J.S., Williams A.J., and Campbell R.W.F. (1995). "Use of 24 h ambulatory ECG recordings in the assessment of new chemical entities in healthy volunteers", *Br J Clin Pharmacol*, 39, 651–656.

Task Force Report of the American Psychiatric Association (1987). *Sudden Death in Psychiatric Patients: TheRole of Neuroleptic Drugs*. American Psychiatric Association, Washington D.C.

Thompson C. (1994). "The use of high–dose antipsychotic medication", *Br J Psychiatry*, 164, 448–458.

Wagstaff A.J., and Bryson H.M. (1995). "Clozapine. A review of its pharmacological properties and therapeutic use in patients with schizophrenia who are unresponsive to or intolerant of classical antipsychotic agents", *CNS Drugs*, 4, 370–400.

Weiden P.J., Dixon L., Frances A., Appelbaum P., Haas G., and Rapkin B. (1991). "Neuroleptic noncompliance in schizophrenia." In *Advances in Neuropsychiatry and Psychopharmacology, Vol. I: Schizophrenia Research* (eds. C.A. Tamminga and S.C. Schulz), Raven Press, New York.

Windgassen K. (1992). "Treatment with neuroleptics: the patient's perspective", *Acta Psychiatr Scand*, 86, 405–410.

Wistedt B., and Palmstierna T. (1991). "Strategies for prevention and treatment of violence by psychotic patients", *Nord J Psychiatry*, 45 (Suppl. 25), 5–11.

9

TREATMENT RESISTANT SCHIZOPHRENIA: A CLINICAL PERSPECTIVE

Bill MacEwan, Sean Flynn and Nathan Schaffer

INTRODUCTION

Schizophrenia is a devastating illness and optimal management can present a challenge for the clinician. This chapter outlines an approach to the clinical management of schizophrenia, with a particular focus on treatment resistant schizophrenia. Clinical vignettes are presented which highlight specific areas where difficulties in treatment can be encountered and which also focus on approaches that our experience has led us to believe are helpful in managing treatment resistant schizophrenia.

THE APPROACH TO TREATMENT RESISTANT SCHIZOPHRENIA

Schizophrenia is a complex and multi-dimensional disorder and the clinical literature clearly demonstrates that treatment response is variable, even in the most straight forward cases. The diversity of clinical response, as well as the uncertain course of illness, has led researchers and clinicians to put forward. several different conceptualizations of treatment resistance. Brenner considered a person with schizophrenia to be treatment resistant if he/she did not return to their pre-morbid level of functioning when treated (Brenner et al., 1990). In our opinion, this definition lacks specificity. In fact, if this rather stringent criterion were applied in general practice, most of those afflicted with schizophrenia could be thought of as displaying treatment resistance as most individuals fail to return to their pre-morbid level of function. This definition also fails to clearly

Schizophrenia: Breaking Down the Barriers. Edited by S.G. Holliday, R.J. Ancill and G.W. MacEwan. © 1996 John Wiley & Sons Ltd

relate the concept of treatment resistance to the specific action of therapeutic agents.

Meltzer considered treatment resistance to be present when any positive symptoms or significant negative symptoms persisted despite treatment (Meltzer, 1990). Again, this definition may be overly general, as specific therapeutic agents may show differential effects. The patient may actually be responsive to the treatments, but the treatment may not be general enough to control all aspects of the disorder.

Kane specifically defined treatment resistance in terms of symptoms that persist after treatment trials of at least three different antipsychotics from at least two different classes which are given for a period of at least six weeks each at a dose of at least 1000 mg of chlorpromazine equivalents (Kane et al., 1988). In our opinion, this is the strongest of the operational definitions as it provides criteria that both have clinical utility and allow for comparisons between different studies.

May offered perhaps the most clinically useful description of the phenomenon of treatment resistance (May et al., 1988). He discussed treatment resistance in terms of a spectrum of treatment response, ranging from the person with schizophrenia whose symptoms completely remit with treatment to one who has profound disturbances of functioning despite intensive treatment, and may require long-term institutionalization.

Depending on which definition of treatment resistance is used, 5 to 25% of schizophrenics may be considered to be resistant to treatment. From a clinical viewpoint, however, it is important to note that the group of persons with treatment resistant schizophrenia is the most difficult to manage for both the short and long term. Persons in this group are much more likely to require costly direct interventions, incur large indirect costs, and suffer from a poor quality of life when compared to treatment responsive schizophrenics. They may be expected to draw more heavily on inpatient hospital resources and to require greater levels of support when maintained in the community.

It is our opinion that this challenging group of patients may hold answers to a number of questions about the mechanisms of schizophrenia. It has long been suspected that resistance to dopamine blocking medications may reflect different underlying pathophysiologic processes in the refractory schizophrenic (Crow, 1980). Thus closer examination of persons who are treatment resistant may help us to more completely understand the complex disorder of schizophrenia.

SYMPTOM RECOGNITION AND DIAGNOSIS

The utility of the concept of treatment resistant schizophrenia ultimately rests on the precision and validity of the diagnostic system. Fortunately standardization of symptom description has improved over the last two decades and today, if the clinician is careful, we can be reasonably sure of our initial diagnoses. Symptom assessment instruments such as the Positive and Negative Syndrome Scale (PANSS) (Kay et al., 1987), the expanded Brief Psychiatric Rating Scale (BBPRS) (Overall and Gorham,1962), and the Scale for Assessment of Positive Symptoms and Scale for Assessment of Negative Symptoms (SAPS and SANS) (Andreasen et al., 1982) all have been useful in grading the severity of patients' symptoms and in allowing cross-study comparisons. Scales that provide measures of functioning, such as the Global Assessment of Functioning (APA, 1994), and those that seek to globally assess the severity of a patient's illness, such as the Clinical Global Impression of Illness (Guy, 1976) are other, complimentary outcomes measures. Perhaps the most useful feature of rating scales is that it allows the clinician to objectively measure the impact of an intervention. Wider acceptance and use of the Diagnostic and Statistical Manual (APA, 1994) may lead to more reliability and validity in the diagnosis of schizophrenia.

In addition to symptom scales, that assess a patient's cross-sectional presentation, clinicians should give careful consideration to the longitudinal course of the illness. The occurrence and degree of mood symptoms are particularly important to assess, as this can help differentiate schizophrenic psychosis from the cross-sectionally similar psychosis often seen in schizoaffective disorder, bipolar disorder, and depression. Despite these advances in symptom scales and diagnostic tools, reconsideration of the diagnosis, even in long-standing and seemingly clear-cut cases, has been shown to be useful. Honer et al., (1994), showed that fully 25% of a large cohort of seemingly "chronic schizophrenic" patients referred to a inpatient unit that specializes in the treatment of refractory schizophrenia, were rediagnosed when strict DSM criteria were used (Honer et al., 1994). The rediagnosis included a thorough review of all available information from past hospitalizations, interviews with family members, medical work-up, symptom inventories, and treatment team consensus, as outlined by Smith (Smith et al., 1992). The new diagnosis arrived at commonly recognized the presence of previously overlooked affective components or medical illnesses that can contribute to the patient's psychosis. When these factors are recognized and co-morbid features appropriately treated, the actual symptoms of schizophrenia tend to improve.

TREATMENT AND RESPONSE MEASUREMENT

Antipsychotic medications remain the primary treatment for schizophrenia. Many patients, however, show little or no benefit from these medications. Collins found that one-half of the patients in a long-stay psychiatric institution who had schizophrenia that showed resistance to treatment were given antipsychotic medications at doses similar to those of patients with acute schizophrenia (Collins et al., 1992). This in itself is an unfortunate situation, but it becomes even more serious when lack of response goes unrecognized or unacknowledged and medications are continued—or even increased—in the face of what are at times marginal benefits. The consensus opinion in the clinical literature is that there appears to be no benefit from increasing dosages of antipsychotics in the treatment resistant schizophrenic group (Rifkin et al., 1992), nor from achieving a higher serum level of medication (Volavki et al., 1992; Shriqui, 1995). Indeed, the high doses of antipsychotics that treatment resistant schizophrenics are often given may increase the short-term side effects and the long-term risks associated with these medications, without a clear clinical benefit to the patient. For these reasons, our general practice is to attempt a decrease in antipsychotic dosages when a patient is admitted to hospital.

There is also a growing suspicion that lack of response to medication may be a general phenomenon, rather that the results of a failure of a particular therapeutic agent. Kinan found that acutely ill schizophrenic and schizoaffective patients who failed to respond to a first trial of antipsychotics were likely to remain unresponsive to a second trial (Kinan et al., 1993). These findings suggests that treatment resistance may be identifiable early in the course of schizophrenia.

THERAPEUTIC OPTIONS: ATYPICAL NEUROLEPTICS

Clozapine

Clozapine has been shown to have improved efficacy over typical antipsychotics in treatment resistant schizophrenia. In double-blind trials comparing clozapine to chlorpromazine, haloperidol, and fluphenazine, clozapine has shown clear advantages (Kane et al., 1988; Pickar et al., 1992). The evidence is particularly robust that clozapine treats positive symptoms better than typical antipsychotics. There remains debate regarding the effect clozapine has on negative symptoms. This focuses on whether the improvements are primarily seen in secondary negative symptoms or, alternatively, as a result of a direct effect on the deficit of primary negative symptoms (Breier et al., 1994). Despite the proven advantage of clozapine in treating treatment resistant schizophrenia, it has been estimated that only 5% of those eligible have received a trial of clozapine (Remington et al., 1996).

One of the notable features of clozapine is that patients treated with it may continue to show improvement after six or more months of treatment (Meltzer, 1990). Brier and others noted that while 18 of 31 patients with refractory schizophrenia responded after one year of clozapine treatment only one of these patients responded after four months of treatment (Brier et al., 1993). The delayed improvement is reported to be particularly marked in the cognitive sphere, in which patients may continue to show improvements for up to twelve months (Carmen et al., 1981). The improvement that clozapine has on tardive dyskinesia may not be apparent for four months or more. Breier et al., suggested that a four month trial is needed to properly assess clozapine response, but that quality of life may continue to improve past the six month mark (Christison et al., 1991).

Risperidone

Risperidone has been shown to be a very effective and well tolerated antipsychotic for patients in the acute phase of schizophrenia (Umbricht and Kane, 1995). Some preliminary evidence suggests that risperidone may also be effective in the treatment resistant schizophrenic group (Lindenmayer et al., 1995; Cavallaro et al., 1995; Keck et al., 1995).

A recently developed and incompletely studied strategy in treatment resistant schizophrenia is augmenting clozapine with low doses of risperidone, a treatment that some clinicians feel can help a subset of patients. Although little is known regarding how these medications act synergistically, competition for metabolism via the hepatic cytochrome P-450 2D6 enzyme system may act to increase clozapine blood levels to a therapeutic level (Tyson et al., 1995). Since a complex and interactive modulation of serotonergic and dopaminergic systems is felt to be responsible for the efficacy of these atypical antipsychotics (Kapur and Remington, 1996), it may be that clozapine and risperidone in combination synergise this modulation.

Side Effects

Extrapyramidal side effects, although rare with clozapine (Umbricht and Kane, 1995) and risperidone (Buchanan, 1995), should not be overlooked. The presence of extrapyramidal syndromes can have both motor and mental effects that may contribute to treatment resistance (Casey, 1994).

COMPLIANCE

The side-effect burden of many psychiatric medications, combined with the lack of insight that so often accompanies the illness, often leads to a lack of compliance to prescribed treatment. For many antipsychotics, serum blood levels are available, although the therapeutic range of most agents is not clear. Nevertheless, blood levels can be useful in determining compliance. Perhaps even more useful in assessing compliance is the use of serum prolactin levels. Three approaches are thought to be useful in dealing with non-compliance. The newer antipsychotics, because of their improved tolerability compared to older drugs, may improve compliance. Long-acting depot antipsychotics simplify treatment protocols, may decrease patients' ambivalence towards treatment, and consequently may improve compliance. A variety of psychosocial interventions, including medication education programs, peer support groups, family education initiatives, and assertive outreach programs all hold promise for improving compliance, although evidence for their efficacy in non-compliance is neither consistent nor robust.

ALTERNATIVE THERAPEUTICS

Other treatments may be used in conjunction with antipsychotic medications. First, a variety of somatic augmentation strategies are available. Benzodiazepines, used in conjunction with antipsychotics, may improve symptoms in up to 50% of schizophrenics (Wolkowitz et al., 1992). Carbamazepine appears to have a beneficial effect in some schizophrenics (Simhandl and Meszaros, 1992). Studies assessing the efficacy of valproate in schizophrenia are somewhat less encouraging (McElroy et al., 1989). The efficacy of lithium augmentation has been similarly questioned. Some studies have shown benefits (Carmen et al., 1981), others little or no benefit (Lerner et al., 1988). Second, electroconvulsvie therapy may improve symptoms when catatonia or affective symptoms are present, but has little or no effect on chronic schizophrenia (Christison et al., 1991). Our experience has been that any of these treatments may benefit certain patients, but that there are few reliable predictors of response. Third, other adjunctive somatic treatments that may be beneficial in some patients include beta-blockers, reserpine, antidepressants, L-dopa, D-amphetamine blockers, calcium channel blockers, and opioids.

There are several simple principles to guide a clinician in the use of adjunctive therapies. (1) Trials of these adjunctive therapies should be undertaken one at a time, last at least four to six weeks, and be aimed at specific target symptoms. (2) When positive symptoms are the target, mood-stabilizers, benozidazpeines, or electronconvulsive therapy may be effective. (3) When negative symptoms are prominent, L-dopa or benzodiazepines can be useful adjuvants. (4) If affective symptoms are present, mood stabilizers, ECT or antidepressants may be beneficial. (5) When impulsivity or aggression are a concern, carbamazepine or propranolol may be useful. (6) In patients with EEG changes, carbamazepine or valproate can be considered.

There is also a wealth of evidence that psycho-social strategies, particularly psychoeducation, family therapy, therapeutic communities, behavioral interventions, and social and occupational rehabilitation programs can have beneficial effects on the overall course of the illness (Falloon and Liberman, 1983; Glynn and Mueser, 1986).

A SYSTEMATIC APPROACH TO CLINICAL MANAGEMENT

The management strategy presented in the following pages is used to guide the management of treatment resistant schizophrenics on a tertiary care psychiatry ward specializing in treatment resistant psychosis. Following admission to the ward, a two-week period of time is used to obtain records of previous treatments, conduct structured psychiatric and psychiatric nurse assessments, and obtain relevant physical assessments, usually including physical examinations, laboratory tests, electroencephalographs, and computerized brain tomography. A social worker completes a birth, developmental, and family history for each patient. Medications are reduced or discontinued when possible. In particular, medications that are not felt to be treating target symptoms are minimized. (When rationalizing medication treatments in this way, it is important to be mindful of the safety of the patient, the staff, and the community.) These assessments are done to gain a comprehensive understanding of the patient, using a bio-psychosocial model. In addition, the data are used in our continuing research efforts.

Following the two week assessment period, a multi-disciplinary diagnostic round is held to establish a DSM-III-R multi-axial diagnosis and to confirm treatment strategies. Once the team has reached the consensus diagnosis as outlined above, we continue treatment of the patient using the algorithm outlined in Figure 1.

Figure 1 displays, in diagram, the general process/procedures that we follow in establishing a diagnosis, determining if a patient is treatment resistant, and initiating a comprehensive treatment regimen. The algorithm begins with the establishment of a diagnosis, as described previously. This process subsumes a variety of issues including general medical status, the natural history of the illness, documentation of response to previous interventions, etc.

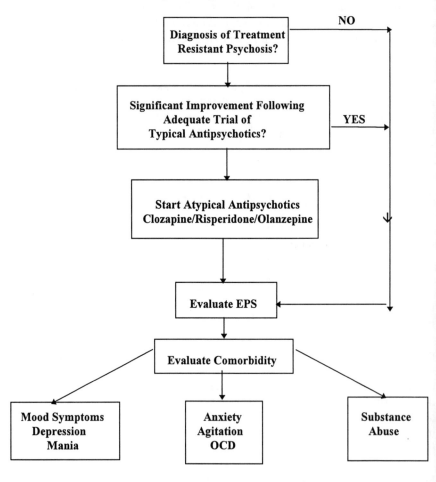

Figure 1.

Following establishment of a valid diagnosis, a decision is made regarding the course of treatment. If the patient has not been given an appropriate course of conventional (typical) antipsychotic medication, such a course is initiated. If an acceptable therapeutic response is achieved, the person, by definition, is not treatment resistant. The person is then given a comprehensive evaluation for the presence of medication side effects and the presence of co-morbid disorders. If present, such disorders are treated and the patient is discharged.

If the patient has a proven record of non-response to adequate trials of medication at appropriate dosage levels, meet the working definition of treatment resistant and is started on an atypical medication—usually clozapine or risperidone.

After a suitable period of time, the patient is re-evaluated to determine if there is a therapeutic response. If the patient responds, he is fully screened for the presence of medication side-effects and for co-morbid disorders. If present, such disorders are treated and the patient is discharged.

If there is no evidence of a therapeutic response, medication is nonetheless continued, as therapeutic effects may emerge only after a longer period of time with atypical antipsychotic agents. At this time, the feasibility of introducing adjunctive therapy is also considered. The person is then evaluatedf or the presence of medication side-effects and of co-morbid disorders. If present, such disorders are treated. The patient is then discharged from hospital and is typically followed as (a) a hospital outpatient, (b) a client of a community mental health team, or (c) a client of a private practice physician.

CLINICAL CASES

The following three cases are presented as examples of how specific patients were managed using the algorithm presented in Figure 1 and described in the previous section. Case One is an example of the addition of clozapine to a treatment regime. Case Two demonstrates the targeting of mood symptoms in a patient with refractory schizophrenia. Case Three demonstrates the treatment of co-morbid obsessive-compulsive symptoms and treatment resistant schizophrenic disorders.

CASE ONE

T.W. was a 25 year old single male Caucasian initially admitted to a provincial psychiatric facility from a boarding home. At the time of his admission to the Refractory Psychosis program he was unemployed and receiving social assistance. Referral was for an assessment regarding refractory psychosis. He had an 8 year history of psychiatric treatment with diagnoses of schizophrenia and a schizoaffective disorder in the past. He had experienced medication trials of trifluoperazine, fluphenazine, loxapine and valproic acid.

Six months prior to admission he had a two month hospitalization with a diagnosis of schizoaffective disorder. He was receiving loxapine 100 mg/day, lithium carbonate 1200 mg/day and benztropine 2 mg/day. Since that time community caregivers had become increasingly concerned about T.W.'s preoccupations, social isolation, and daily auditory hallucinations which commented on his behavior and called him names. As well he was reporting that an entity was both touching his face and using people at the boarding home to control him.

Review of his history indicated that his mother was diagnosed with and treated for paranoid schizophrenia. He also had a fraternal twin who was chronically hospitalized for treatment of schizophrenia and a sister who was diagnosed with a bipolar mood disorder. There were no birth complications and he was described as being a shy and quiet child who did well in school. He experimented with drugs in high-school but did not have a substance abuse pattern and remained a casual social drinker. His highest occupational functioning occurred following completion of high school when he worked as a photo lab technician for six months. He did not report a history of sexual abuse, and had a heterosexual orientation. Although he was not in an intimate relationship, he did have one in his late teens.

At age 20, T.W. began feeling disconnected from others and reported having experiences of time being lengthened and of noticing strange coincidences. At that time his mother abandoned the family home and he became increasingly withdrawn, exhibiting over-sleeping, and reporting feelings of hopelessness. After a few months he began feeling both that he had telepathic powers and that others could read his mind. He then became paranoid, hearing whispers giving him orders. He was subsequently hospitalized for five months and was diagnosed with an acute schizophrenic episode that improved on trifluoperazine 7 mg/day and benztropine 2 mg/day.

Since then he has been hospitalized on nine occasions for treatment of psychosis with symptoms including auditory hallucinations, persecutory delusions, ideas of reference, thought withdrawal and insertion and aggression. He has been treated with neuroleptics, mostly trifluoperazine by itself and in combination with loxapine or valproic acid, and more recently loxapine with lithium carbonate. His relapses occurred both in context of compliance and noncompliance with medications. He was felt to have been almost continuously psychotic, experiencing chronic auditory hallucinations. He was a smoker but did not have any significant medical problems.

On his admission mental status examination, he was noted to be accessible and oriented. He had mild lateral jaw movements but his speech was unaffected. Mood and affect were euthymic with a reasonable range. He was experiencing multiple auditory hallucinations that were commenting and criticizing, and he was also talking about an entity touching his face as previously described. He had insight into having a mental illness and was agreeable to hospitalization. He scored 30/30 on the Mini Mental-State Examination (MMSE) and he had an admission PANSS total score of 64 with a positive subscale of 14, negative subscale of 17, and a general psychopathology subscale of 33.

His physical examination was unremarkable except for the aforementioned movement disorder. Admission blood work was normal and his lithium level was 0.7 mmol/L.

T.W.'s file was reviewed in detail during a multidisciplinary diagnostic round and his DSM-III-R multi-axial diagnoses included:

Axis 1   Schizophrenia, paranoid, stable-chronic with acute exacerbation,
                Major depression in remission.
Axis II   No diagnosis
Axis III   Early tardive dyskinesia
Axis IV   Mild stressors
Axis V   GAF admission 25; GAF best in past year 35

The treatment team concluded that a diagnosis of schizoaffective disorder was not warranted since, although he had mood lability, he had never met the criteria for a manic episode and his two depressive episodes were of a relatively short duration.

In terms of the Figure 1 flowchart, he had a well-established diagnosis of schizophrenia and well-documented failure of trials of typical anti-psychotic agents, both alone and with augmentation. He was determined to meet the criteria for treatment resistant schizophrenia and a decision was made to take the next step of starting a trial of an atypical antipsychotic agent.

It was decided, on the basis of his presentation, that he would be a good clozapine candidate and informed consent was obtained for treatment with clozapine. He had an exacerbation of his psychotic symptoms when being changed over from loxapine to clozapine, but these settled with increased clozapine doses of 300 mg/day. Throughout the switch he remained on lithium. After six weeks of hospitalization, it was determined that he was tolerating his medication well and was free of hallucinations or paranoia. He was having less thought disorganization, was more interactive and had improved volition. His discharge PANSS total score was 43: positive subscale of 19, negative subscale of 11 and a general psychopathology subscale of 23.

Evaluation of medication side effects indicated that he was also having reduced dyskinesia. In keeping with Figure 1, it was also determined that his co-morbid mood disorder was also well managed with lithium.

T.W. was then discharged to a boarding home with mental health team follow-up and it was felt the role of lithium could be reconsidered in the future, using a challenge/rechallenge approach in a time of relative stability of symptoms.

CASE TWO

A.M. was a 36 year old, single unemployed male who was living in his own apartment and was on social assistance. He was initially admitted to a provincial psychiatric facility following referral by a community mental health team for an assessment of a potentially refractory psychosis. At time of referral he was taking loxapine 100 mg/day, carbamazepine 900 mg/day and clonazepam 2 mg/day, but despite this was deteriorating and becoming more inappropriate in his behaviour. He was having thought disorganization as well as withdrawal, the latter related to paranoid delusions that the CIA were after him and were trying to brainwash him. His mood was also mildly elevated and he dressed more flamboyantly than usual.

Review of his family history indicated that his father had been treated with antipsychotic medication, possibly for a bipolar mood disorder, and that his younger brother was mentally handicapped. A.M.'s medical history was significant for heavy smoking and he did have a history of episodic alcohol abuse and currently was using alcohol more regularly It was felt that the alcohol use may have been due to his deterioration. He did not abuse street drugs. His birth was uncomplicated and at term, but his mother was treated for hypertension in the latter two weeks of the pregnancy. Developmental milestones were normal. His father, an engineer, was often away from home and their relationship was never close. His mother, a retired nurse, was his primary caregiver. His parents divorced when he was ten, and he lived with his mother. He was an average student. He was not very social but usually had a close friend. He quit school in grade 10 but later returned and obtained a high school diploma. He worked sporadically as a waiter and taxi driver. He had one long-term heterosexual relationship in his early 30s that has since ended.

A.M. experienced a brief psychosis in the context of hashish abuse at age 16. His first formal psychiatric contact was at age 18, when he was seen as an outpatient regarding sexual identity concerns. He was hospitalized for the first time at age 22. This occurred when, after being was charged with common assault, he was diagnosed with catatonic schizophrenia and spent 2.5 months in a forensic facility. At age 29, he was rehospitalized following an assault on his father. At that time his mental status examination revealed grandiose and persecutory delusions and the presence of a thought disorder. Treatment was initiated for paranoid schizophrenia and obsessive-compulsive personality traits. He was administered haloperidol which was later switched to depot pipothiazine palmitate prior to discharge. At age 35, he had a third admission to hospital following an incident in which he disrobed in public. On examination he was noted to be irritable with blunted and inappropriate affect, posturing and a thought disorder. His discharge diagnosis was schizoaffective disorder and he was treated with loxapine, carbamazepine and clonazepam.

Since that last admision and in the period prior to and leading up to his referral he had been treated with trifluoperazine, pimozide, flupenthixol, haloperidol, pipotiazine, lithium and carbamazepine. There was a consensus among his care-givers, however, that his response to those agents had been suboptimal.

On his admission mental status, he was noted to be rather oddly dressed in brightly coloured but uncoordinated colors and inappropriately warm clothing. He was detached and aloof and he tended to answer sarcastically. He was also guarded, and his thought processes were circumstantial, occasionally loose, and characterized by a pseudophilosophical style. He reported a paranoid delusion regarding the CIA. He denied hallucinations. He had bizarre and concrete proverb interpretation. His vocabulary was good, but his judgment was impaired and he had only minimal insight into his illness. He scored 30/30 on the MMSE and his admission PANSS total score was 101, with a positive subscale of 24, a negative subscale of 27 and a general psychopathology subscale of 50.

His physical examination was unremarkable and he had normal routine blood work including a negative HIV screen done at his request. EKG, CXR and a non-contrast head CT were non-contributory.

During the early stages of his admission, collateral information was obtained and his file was reviewed in detail during a multidisciplinary diagnostic round. His DSM-III-R multi-axial diagnoses included:

Axis 1   Schizophrenia, undifferentiated, chronic with acute exacerbation; alcohol abuse
Axis 2   Narcissistic, histrionic traits
Axis 3   None
Axis 4   Mild; family conflict
Axis 5   Current 25; highest in past year—30

It was determined at the diagnostic rounds that he did not satisfy DSM-III-R criteria for schizoaffective disorder, as the mood symptoms did not seem to form a major component of his illness, although he did have a history of affective lability.

In terms of the Figure 1 flowchart, he had a well-established diagnosis of schizophrenia and well-documented failure of trials of typical anti-psychotic agents, both alone and with augmentation. He was found to meet the criteria for treatment resistant schizophrenia and a decision was made to take the next step of starting a trial of an atypical antipsychotic agent.

It was felt he would be a good clozapine candidate. Therefore, his carbamazepine was discontinued and he was started on clozapine in a cross-over fashion in which his clonazepam and loxapine were gradually tapered and his clozapine titrated upwards. He physically tolerated this well with only minimal sedation but he did have mild deterioration in his mental state. He was reviewed again by his caregivers including his community psychiatrist after six weeks on clozapine when his dose was 525 mg/day.

In terms of the Figure 1 flowchart, at this time A.M. was also evaluated for the presence of side effects and for the treatment of co-morbid disorders. His side effect profile was unremarkable. However, his overall condition was felt to be little changed from admission. Given the established mood features, it was decided to begin valproic acid as an augmentation strategy. This treatment proved effective and after about 2–3 weeks considerable improvement was noted and he was found to be less thought disordered and more organized.

He was subsequently discharged to his apartment with follow up arranged through a local mental health team. Upon discharge his PANSS was repeated and his total score was 61 with a positive subscale of 14, a negative subscale of 18 and a general psychopathology subscale of 29.

CASE THREE

R.S. was an 18 year old single male Caucasian admitted electively for assessment of treatment-psychosis. At the time of his admission he was residing with a foster family. He had had ongoing problems since childhood and had his first psychiatric contact at age four–for behavioral problems in context of his parents marital discord. He had been under psychiatric care on a continuous basis since age 12. At that time he was reported to have significant conduct problems, to be hearing voices, and to be experiencing paranoid delusions as well as disorganized thoughts. On admission, his main concern was the presence of intrusive, unwanted thoughts which at times would take form of a song going round and round in his mind. He also reported periodically experiencing sensations of panic as well as episodes of losing his concentration, having difficulty moving and associated palpitations. His history included reports of occasional inappropriate behavior consisting of loud laughter for no apparent reason.

On admission it was established that he had been taking risperidone 6 mg/day for a number of months and that this had helped eliminate the intermittent auditory hallucinations. There was no recent or past history of alcohol or illicit drug abuse. He had no significant medical concerns.

Review of his family history revealed that both his mother and maternal grandmother had experienced depression, while his older brother had been identified as having a conduct disorder. He also had a first cousin with agoraphobia. There were no significant birth complications and the family reported normal developmental milestones. His father was a miner who was physically abusive. His mother worked as a parking lot attendant and was more nurturing. As a toddler he was noted to be odd and isolative and had to repeat kindergarten. In school, he had difficulty sustaining attention and was in special education for grades 3–4. At age 10, he had his IQ tested as 92. He had been living with the same foster parents since age nine when his parents finally separated.

Following his first psychiatric admission he had four additional hospitalizations with a variety of diagnoses including conduct disorder, schizophrenia, obsessive-compulsive disorder, and atypical pervasive developmental disorder. Past treatments included chlorpromazine, haloperidol (up to 60 mg/day for six months) and trifluoperazine. He has also had medication-free periods in which he became clearly psychotic with disorganization and command hallucinations. He also had a trial of clozapine with dosages up to 400 mg/day, but developed granulocytopenia necessitating discontinuation. He had also had augmentation trials with paroxetine and valproic acid.

On admission his mental status examination revealed him to be well groomed, and pleasant. Rapport was good but he had difficulty elaborating on the nature of his symptoms. His affect was bright and he exhibited occasional inappropriate smiling. He reported feeling euthymic. His thought content was remarkable for the presence of intrusive thoughts and music, together with feelings of panic. He had a moderate degree of insight into his condition. The PANSS total was 83; 17 positive, 20 negative, 46 general.

Physical examination and routine blood work were unremarkable. CT scan showed mild to moderate cerebral tissue loss with sulcal prominence particularly in the parietal regions. His EEG while awake and drowsy, was normal. Neuropsychological testing showed normal range of functioning and normal IQ.

In the initial stages of his admission, old records and ward observations were reviewed in detail and his case presented at multidisciplinary diagnostic rounds. His DSM-III-R multi-axial diagnoses included:

Axis I   Schizophrenia, chronic, residual
          ? Panic disorder/OCD
Axis II   None
Axis III Resolved granulocytopenia secondary to clozapine
Axis IV   Moderate
Axis V   GAF admission 35; GAF best in past year 43

In terms of the Figure 1 flowchart, he had a well-established diagnosis of schizophrenia and well-documented failure of trials of typical anti-psychotic agents, both alone and with augmentation. He was found to meet the criteria for treatment resistant schizophrenia and a decision was made to take the next step of starting a trial of an atypical antipsychotic agent. He was also noted be experiencing several co-morbid problems.

Given his previous history with clozapine, and his partial response to risperidone, it was decided to continue risperidone. In terms of the Figure 1 flowchart, since the antipsychotic treatment was well established, the next focus was upon his co-morbid disorders. It was then decided that a trial of augmentation with clomipramine would also be initiated. This augmentation strategy was begun but after two weeks when his dose was 50 mg/d it was discontinued due to worsening of his symptoms. It was then decided to try low dose clonazepam (0.5 mg/day). He then showed significant improvement in that his intrusive thoughts were less problematic for him and he was no longer having episodes of experiencing feelings of panic. Evaluation of the side effects of medication proved to be unremarkable and there remained no major behavioral concerns except for ongoing social isolation. He was then discharged back to the community after five weeks in hospital. Discharge PANSS was 65 total (13 positive, 15 negative and 37 general).

SUMMARY

This chapter has focused upon treatment resistant schizophrenia from a clinical perspective. We have attempted to provide an overview of treatment resistant schizophrenia which emphasizes the clinical approach we have taken when assessing and treating patients who exhibit a treatment resistant psychosis.

The foundation of the clinical program is the standardized clinical assessment of a patient's history and current presentation. This allows the treatment team to reach a diagnosis by team consensus. The team then focuses on the dominant diagnosis (in the case of comorbid diagnoses) or dominant symptoms. Often the patient's psychotic symptoms predominate, so after establishing a degree of improvement on an antipsychotic the team then moves on to identify and treat the next most prominent symptoms. This step by step approach, which was illustrated and discussed in the previous sections of the chapter, provides a rationale for action in the common situations in which a patient with a multiplicity of symptoms is treated with a number of medications.

In Case One, the patient's prominent problem was refractory psychosis. There was also a history of mood lability which had demonstrated some improvement on lithium. After stabilizing the psychosis with clozapine, the mood lability was managed through the use of lithium. The overall effect was a significant degree of improvement.

In Case Two, the patient had prominent refractory psychosis which improved on treatment with clozapine but did not resolve to a satisfactory degree. Because of the patient's past history of mood problems, a trial of valproic acid was added with the effect of obtaining a significant remission of his symptoms.

In Case Three, the patient presented a refractory schizophrenia with comorbid diagnoses of panic disorder and OCD. A history of granulocytopenia while on clozapine dictated a trial of risperidone. The improvement on risperidone was not satisfactory so his comorbid diagnoses were treated, ultimately with clonazepam, while maintaining his treatment with risperidone. This strategy resulted in significant improvement.

The final aspect of our treatment approach is to fully reassess all of our patients who have not improved enough. In all three case examples each patient had significant improvement but was still ill at time of discharge. We work with outpatient services and community mental health teams to maintain the level of improvement achieved in hospital. We then readmit patients who have relapsed or who are identified as needing further trials of medications. These patients are fully reassessed to determine if their symptom presentation and diagnoses are consistent with previous assessment.

ACKNOWLEDGEMENTS

The authors would like to thank Dr. Lonn Myronuk for his help with literature research and Tracey Davies for her secretarial support.

REFERENCES

Andreasen N.C., and Olsen S. (1982) Negative vs Positive Schizophrenia: Definition and Validation, *Archives of General Psychiatry*, 39, 789–794.

Diagnostic and Statistical Manual of Mental Disorders, 4th Edition (1994), American Psychiatric Association , Washington, DC.

Breier A., Buchanan R.W., Kirkpatrick B., Davis O.R., Irish D., Summerfelt A., Carpenter W.T. (1994) Effects of Clozapine on Positive and Negative Symptoms in Outpatients with Schizophrenia, *American Journal of Psychiatry*, 151, 20–26.

Brenner H.D. et al. (1990) Defining Treatment of Refractoriness in Schizophrenia, *Schizophrenia Bulletin*, 16(4), 551–561.

Brier A. et al. (1993) Clozapine Treatment of Outpatients with Schizophrenia, 2: Outcomes and Long–term response patterns, *Hospital and Community Psychiatry*, 44, 1145–1149.

Buchanan R.W. (1995) Clozapine: Efficacy and Safety, *Schizophrenia Bulletin*, 21, 4, 579–591.

Carmen J.S., Bigelow L.B., and Wyatt R..J. (1981) Lithium Combined with Neuroleptics in Chronic Schizophrenia and Schizoaffective Patients, *Journal of Clinical Psychiatry*, 42: 124–128.

Casey D.E. (1994) Motor and Mental Aspects of Acute Extrapyramidal Syndromes, *Acta Psychiatr Scand*, 89(Suppl 380), 14–20.

Cavallaro R., Colombo C., and Smeraldi E. (1995) A Pilot, Open Study on the Treatment of Refractory Schizophrenia with Risperidone and Clozapine, *Human Psychopharmacology*, 10, 231–234.

Christison G.W., Kirch D.G. and Wyatt R.,J. (1991) Choosing Among Alternative Somatic Treatments for Schizophrenia, *Schizophrenia Bulletin*, 17(2), 217–245.

Collins E.J., Hogan T. and Awad A.G. (1992) The Pharmacoepidemiology of Treatment Resistant Schizophrenia, *Canadian Journal of Psychiatry*, 37(4), 192–195.

Crow T.,J. (1980) Molecular Pathology of Schizophrenia: More than One Disease Process?, *British Medical Journal*, 280, 1–9.

Falloon I.R.H. and Liberman R. (1983) *Interactions Between Drug and Psychosocial Therapy in Schizophrenia*, *Schizophrenia Bulletin*, 9, 543–554.

Glynn S. and Mueser K.T. (1986) Social Learning for Chronic Mental Inpatients, *Schizophrenia Bulletin*, 12, 648–668.

Guy W. (1976) ECDEU *Assessment Manual for Psychopharmacology*, *Revised* (Publication ADM 76–338), Rockville Pike, MD: US Department of Health, Education, and Welfare.

Higenbottam J (1994) Treating Schizophrenia: Psychosocial Interventions, *British Columbia Medical Journal*, 36(7), 472–474.

Honer, W.G. et al., (1994) Diagnostic Reassessment and Treatment Response in Schizophrenia, *Journal of Clinical Psychiatry*, 55, 528–532.

Kane J., Honigfeld G., Singer J. and Meltzer H. (1988) Clozapine for the Treatment Resistant Schizophrenic; A Double–Blind Comparison with Chlorpromazine, *Archives of General Psychiatry*, 45, 789–796.

Kane, J. et al., (1988) Clozapine for the Treatment–Resistant Schizophrenic: A Double–Blind Comparison with Chlorpromazine/Benztropine, *Archives of General Psychiatry*, 45, 789–796.

Kapur S., Remington G. (1996) *Serotonin–Dopamine Interaction and Its Relevance to Schizophrenia*, *American Journal of Psychiatry*, 153(4), 466–476.

Kay S., Fiszbein and Opler L.A. (1987) The Positive and Negative Syndrome Scale (PANSS) for Schizophrenia, *Schizophrenia Bulletin*, 13, 261–276.

Keck P.E., Wilson D.R., Strakowski S.M., McElroy S.L., Kizer D.L., Balitreri T.M., Holtman H.M., DePrirst M. (1995) Clinical Predictors of Acute Risperidone Response in Schizophrenia, Schizoaffective Disorder and Psychotic Mood Disorders, *Journal of Clinical Psychiatry,* 56(10), 466–470.

Kinan B.J., Kiane J.M., Johns C., Perovich R., Ismai M, Koren A., Widen (1993) Treatment of Neuroleptic–resistant Schizophrenic Relapse, *Psychopharmacology Bulletin,* 29, 309–314.

Lerner Y., Mintzer Y., and Shestatsky M. (1988) Lithium Combined with Haloperidol in Schizophrenic Patients, *British Journal of Psychiatry,* 153, 359–362.

Lindenmayer J.P. et al., (1995) *Use of Risperidone in Neuroleptic Refractory Schizophrenics in a State Psychiatric Center,* New Research Program and Abstracts of the 148th Annual Meeting of the American Psychiatric Association; May 23, 1995; Miami, Florida. Abstract NR228:117.

May, et al., (1988) *A Systematic Approach to Treatment Resistance in Schizophrenic Disorders, Treatment Resistance in Schizophrenia* (Ed. S. Dencker and F. Kulhanek), Vieweg, Braunschweig/Weisbaden, 22–33.

McElroy S.L. et al., (1989) Valproate in Psychiatric Disorders: Literature Review and Clinical Guidelines, *Journal of Clinical Psychiatry,* 50(Suppl.3), 23–29.

Meltzer H.Y. et al., (1990) Effects of Six Months of Clozapine Treatment on the Quality of Life of Chronic Schizophrenic Patients, *Hospital and Community Psychiatry,* 41, 892–897.

Meltzer, H.Y. (1990). Commentary: Defining Treatment Refractoriness in Schizophrenia *Schizophrenia Bulletin,* 16(4), 563–565.

Overall J.E. and Gorham D.R. (1962) The Brief Psychiatric Rating Scale, *Psychological Reports,* 10, 799–812.

Pickar D., Owen R.R., Litman R.E., Konicki E., Gutierrez R., Rapaport M.H. (1992) Clinical and Biological Response to Clozapine in Patients with Schizophrenia: Cross Over Comparison with Fluphenazine, *Archives of General Psychiatry,* 49, 345–353.

Remington G.J. et al., (1996) Clozapine: Current Status and Role in the Pharmacotherapy of Schizophrenia, *Canadian Journal of Psychiatry,* 41, 161–166.

Rifkin A., Doddi S., Karajgi B., Borenstein M., Wachpress M. (1991) Dosage of Haloperidol for Schizophrenia, *Archives of General psychiatry,* 48, 166–170.

Shriqui C.L. Neuroleptic Dosing and Neuroleptic Plasma Levels in Schizophrenia Determining the Optimal Regimen, *Canadian Journal of Psychiatry,* 40:9(Suppl.2), 38–48.

Simhandl C. and Meszaros K. (1992) The use of Carbamazepine in the Treatment of Schizophrenic and Schizoaffective Psychoses: A Review, *Journal of Psychiatry and Neuroscience*, 17, 1–14.

Smith G.N. et al., (1992) Diagnostic Confusion in Treatment–refractory Psychotic Patients, *Journal of Clinical Psychiatry*, 53, 197–200.

Tyson S.C., Devane C.L. and Risch S.C. (1995) Pharmacokinetic Interaction Between Risperidone and Clozapine, *American Journal of Psychiatry*, 152(9), 1401–1402.

Umbbricht D., Kane J.M. (1995) Risperidone: Efficacy and Safety, *Schizophrenia Bulletin*, 21(11), 593–606.

Volavka J., Cooper T., Czobboi P., Bitter I., Melisner M., Laska E., Gastanaga, Doryan R. (1992) Haloperidol Blood Levels and Clinical Effects, *Archives of General Ppsychiatry*, 49, 354–361.

Wolkowitz O.M. et al., (1992) Benzodiazepine Augmentation of Neuroleptics in Treatment–Resistant Schizophrenia, *Psychopharmacology Bulletin*, 28(3), 291–295.

10

PRECLINICAL PROFILE OF SEROQUEL (QUETIAPINE): AN ATYPICAL ANTIPSYCHOTIC WITH CLOZAPINE-LIKE PHARMACOLOGY

JEFFREY M. GOLDSTEIN

INTRODUCTION

For many years, research scientists have tried to extend the understanding of schizophrenia beyond the dopaminergic hypothesis because it does not fully explain the pathogenesis and etiology of the illness. However, the hypothesis remains appealing because the linkage between dopaminergic systems and schizophrenia seems to be demonstrable through experimentation. Briefly, this theory proposes that schizophrenia is due to a hyperactivity in dopaminergic systems in critical brain regions (e.g., the nucleus accumbens and other limbic system areas). This hypothesis evolved primarily because all known antipsychotic agents are dopaminergic receptor antagonists, and agents that mimic or enhance the activity of dopamine (DA) at postsynaptic receptor sites (e.g., amphetamine) have precipitated psychotic episodes in humans.

The methods used to evaluate the antipsychotic potential of experimental agents in animals have remained essentially the same since the introduction of chlorpromazine in the 1950s. Neuropharmacologists have developed more highly sophisticated methods for evaluating the antagonism of the activities of dopaminergic agonists by antipsychotic drugs, but these procedures are still measuring the same end point (i.e., dopaminergic receptor blockade).

Schizophrenia: Breaking Down the Barriers. Edited by S.G. Holliday, R.J. Ancill and G.W. MacEwan. © 1996 John Wiley & Sons Ltd

Thus, for the most part, the procedures that have been developed and which have been routinely used to discover and evaluate antipsychotic agents have been based on the antagonism of the effects of either indirect-acting (e.g., amphetamine) or direct-acting (e.g., apomorphine) DA agonists (i.e., an antagonism of DA-mediated effects) (Worms et al., 1983). One of the few classical procedures used to predict antipsychotic activity that does not depend upon the antagonism of the effects of DA agonists is the conditioned avoidance procedure; however, the mechanism of action of antipsychotic drugs in this procedure is still believed to be via a dopaminergic receptor blockade.

The problem with these tests, which are mostly based on measures of dopamine antagonist effects, is that they ultimately lead to the discovery of haloperidol-like drugs—drugs that are associated with side effects in humans. The strategy for drug development adopted by Zeneca Pharmaceuticals was based on measurements that were more likely to predict a clozapine-like agent. Such drugs have a low DA D_2 receptor affinity and higher serotonin 5-HT2 receptor affinity (clozapine-like binding ratio), low catalepsy potential, selective effects on mesolimbic A10 DA cells, and low dystonic liability in haloperidol-sensitized and drug-naive monkeys. These were a few of the key measures that formed the antipsychotic project screening process. As a result of these endeavors, quetiapine was discovered in 1984 in the Wilmington, Delaware laboratories of Zeneca (formerly ICI) Pharmaceuticals.

This chapter provides a review of the pharmacologic profile of quetiapine as it has been developed based on behavioral, electrophysiological, and neurochemical tests designed to predict antipsychotic activity and liability for EPS and TD. The tests have been performed in multiple species following acute and chronic administration of quetiapine and comparator agents. Evaluations included the following: (a) conditioned avoidance tests in squirrel monkeys, tests to determine drug effects in haloperidol-sensitized and drug-naive Cebus monkeys, and tests of behavioral paradigms using apomorphine-and amphetamine-induced behavioral alterations; (b) electrophysiologic tests measuring either reversal of DA agonist-induced inhibition of DA cell firing or effects on spontaneous activity of DA cells; and (c) neurochemical studies measuring receptor binding and indices of DA receptor blockade and metabolism. Additional studies reviewed here and published by investigators external to Zeneca Pharmaceuticals provided further evidence of clozapine-like properties for quetiapine.

. EVALUATION OF QUETIAPINE IN TESTS PREDICTIVE OF ANTIPSYCHOTIC EFFECTS

.1 CONDITIONED AVOIDANCE TEST IN SQUIRREL MONKEYS

The conditioned avoidance response (CAR) paradigm, a classic procedure for detecting and evaluating antipsychotic agents, was performed in squirrel monkeys to yield data more relevant to humans.

The dose–response curves for quetiapine and reference agents are graphically presented in Figure 1. Quetiapine produced dose-related inhibition of CAR in squirrel monkeys. $ED_{50}s$ (doses producing 50% inhibition of CAR) were found to be 0.30, 2.9, 10.5, and 23.8 mg/kg p.o. for haloperidol, chlorpromazine, quetiapine, and clozapine, respectively. Although quetiapine was less potent than either haloperidol or chlorpromazine, it was approximately 2.3 times more potent than clozapine in this procedure.

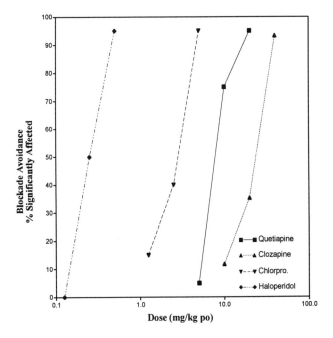

* n = 15 to 20 monkeys per treatment group

Figure 1.. Effect of Quetiapine, Clozapine, Chlorpromazine, and Haloperidol on Conditioned Avoidance in Squirrel Monkeys*

1.2 APOMORPHINE-INDUCED BLINKING TEST IN SQUIRREL MONKEYS

Apomorphine has been shown to dramatically increase the eyeblink rate in squirrel monkeys (Migler et al., 1993). This finding was of interest as schizophrenics have been reported to have an elevated rate of blinking (Stevens, 1978; Karson et al., 1981). Furthermore, standard antipsychotic agents (i.e., chlorpromazine or pimozide) antagonize this effect in squirrel monkeys. Thus, the antagonism of apomorphine-induced blinking in the squirrel monkey test has been used as a second test for the prediction of potential antipsychotic activity.

Quetiapine and chlorpromazine at doses of 2.5 mg/kg p.o. were approximately equal in antagonizing apomorphine-induced blinking, exhibiting a 46% and 50% decrease in blinking, respectively (ED50s = 2.1 and 1.7 mg/kg p.o.). Clozapine produced a comparable decrease at 10 mg/kg p.o., with an ED_{50} of 7.7 mg/kg p.o.. Quetiapine was approximately 3.7 times as potent as clozapine.

1.3 APOMORPHINE-INDUCED VISUAL SEARCHING IN CATS

The cat was chosen because DA agonists, (i.e., amphetamine) has been shown to produce a significant increase in visual searching in this species (Ellinwood and Sudilovsky, 1973). Apomorphine, a direct-acting DA agonist, was used instead of amphetamine, which as an indirect-acting agent is less specific. Apomorphine elicited a significant, dose-related increase in visual searching behavior that could be antagonized by reference antipsychotic agents.

Quetiapine produced a dose-related antagonism of apomorphine-induced visual searching in cats. The minimal effective doses (MEDs) (i.e., the lowest dose of drug producing a statistically significant decrease in the number of searches elicited by subsequent apomorphine administration) were 0.62, 2.5, and 5 mg/kg p.o., respectively, for chlorpromazine, quetiapine, and clozapine. Based on its MED, the potency of quetiapine was approximately twice that of clozapine. Furthermore, quetiapine produced a greater magnitude of effect than clozapine as an antagonist of apomorphine-induced searching in cats.

1.4 NORMALIZATION OF APOMORPHINE INDUCED ACTIVITY IN MICE

Clinically effective antipsychotic drugs have been reported to antagonize apomorphine-induced climbing in mice (Martres et al., 1977). Since all clinically effective antipsychotic agents significantly antagonize climbing, this test was selected as one of our primary behavioral tests for antipsychotic potential. The major weakness of the test is that several psychotropic agents that are not antipsychotics also antagonize the climbing response—unfortunately at moderate doses (Simpson et al., 1976; Gulmann et al., 1976).To overcome this difficulty, a new test, the apomorphine swimming normalization test, was developed (Migler et al., 1993).This second test is performed immediately after the climbing test. The mice are removed from the climbing cages and placed for 2 minutes in a doughnut-shaped tank with the water at room temperature. The number of 180 degree laps around the tank is counted. Untreated-or vehicle-treated mice swim and produce a median score of approximately 20 180 degree laps, while apomorphine-treated mice generally score a median of zero. All known clinically effective antipsychotic drugs that have been tested prevent this behavioral disruption and normalize behavior. The reinstitution of normal swimming behavior is a unique feature of this procedure and allows for the elimination of nonspecific sedatives that show up in other tests as false positives (e.g., apomorphine-induced climbing). Other psychotropic drugs that are not antipsychotic agents but which antagonize climbing (propranolol, diazepam, amitriptyline, mianserin, promethazine, phenoxybenzamine, arecoline, yohimbine, and physostigmine) are generally also inactive in this test. Thus, the apomorphine swimming normalization test is considered more predictive of antipsychotic activity in humans than the climbing test because it detects fewer false positives.

Migler et al (1993) found that quetiapine and clozapine antagonized apomorphine-induced climbing in a dose-related manner; however, both drugs were only weakly active, exhibiting MEDs of 80 mg/kg and 40 mg/kg p.o., respectively. In addition, quetiapine and clozapine both caused significant, dose-related increases in swimming, and they were approximately equal in potency in that they both exhibited MEDs of 40 mg/kg PO (Table 1). Thus, quetiapine exhibits potential antipsychotic activity in these tests, and although it is approximately one-half as potent as clozapine in the climbing procedure, it is approximately equipotent compared to clozapine in the apomorphine swimming normalization procedure.

Table 1. **Activity of Quetiapine and Clozapine in the Apomorphine-Induced Climbing and Apomorphine Swimming Normalization Test in Mice**

Treatment	Dose (mg/kg PO)	Mean Climbing Score			p-Value*	Median Swimming Score	p-Value*
Vehicle	--	18.5	±	2.4		0	
Quetiapine	10	19.9	±	2.1	NS#	0	NS
	20	18.8	±	2.4	NS	0	NS
	40	14.9	±	2.8	NS	8	p < 0.01
	80	7.8	±	2.7	p < 0.01	20	p < 0.01
Clozapine	10	22.8	±	2.2	NS	0.5	NS
	20	19.5	±	2.7	NS	1.5	NS
	40	5.1	±	2.2	p < 0.01	13.5	p < 0.01
	80	0.1	±	0.1	p < 0.01	15.5	p < 0.01

* Determined by Student's t-test (two tailed) comparing drug-treated to vehicle-treated control. n = 20 mice per treatment group
# NS - Not significantly different from vehicle, p > 0.05

1.5 AMPHETAMINE SWIMMING NORMALIZATION TEST IN MICE

A second normalization test, the amphetamine swimming normalization test in mice, is also a new tool for determining antipsychotic effect of drugs (Migler et al., 1993). In this test, the agent that induces the disruption of swimming is amphetamine, a compound that is known to produce psychotomimetic effects in humans. In this respect, the amphetamine swimming normalization test may be more predictive of this potential for antipsychotic effects than the apomorphine swimming normalization test, since apomorphine has not been reported to have psychotomimetic effects in humans. In the amphetamine swimming normalization test, the magnitude of effect of clozapine is comparable with that of other antipsychotic agents and significant effects with clozapine have been noted at about half the dose required in the apomorphine normalization test. For this reason, the test is considered to be sensitive to the effects of antipsychotic agents.

The swimming of mice treated only with vehicle (i.p. or p.o.) was completely blocked by amphetamine at a dose of 2.5 mg/kg i.p.. Swimming was restored (i.e., "normalized") in a dose-related manner by quetiapine, clozapine, and chlorpromazine. The magnitude of effect (e.g. maximal increase in swimming scores) of the three agents was comparable. Chlorpromazine was found to be more potent than clozapine, which is a reflection of their reported clinical order of potency. Although quetiapine was found somewhat less potent than clozapine after p.o. administration, the two agents were approximately equipotent following i.p. administration.

1.6 AMPHETAMINE-INDUCED HYPERACTIVITY IN RATS

The antagonism of amphetamine-induced hyperactivity test in rats is a widely used procedure for detecting potential antipsychotic agents. Quetiapine, clozapine, and fluperlapine all produced a dose-related decrease in amphetamine hyperactivity. Based on the $ED_{50}s$, quetiapine (ED_{50}=50 mg/kg PO) was less potent than either clozapine or fluperlapine ($ED_{50}s$=12.2 and 16.2 mg/kg PO, respectively) in this test.

2. EVALUATION OF QUETIAPINE IN TESTS PREDICTIVE OF EXTRAPYRAMIDAL SIDE EFFECTS

2.1 QUETIAPINE VS. REFERENCE ANTIPSYCHOTICS IN CEBUS MONKEYS

Cebus monkeys treated with haloperidol (1 mg/kg p.o., once per week) eventually develop dyskinetic reactions that resemble TD (Weiss et al., 1977; Casey et al., 1980; Casey, 1995). This effect is referred to as "sensitization". The reactions observed in sensitized monkeys include oral reactions (tongue protrusions, opening and closing of the mouth, chewing on hands or feet, and licking or biting the bars of the cage) and/or dyskinetic reactions, consisting of jerking the arms or legs and twisting of the trunk or neck.

The reactions in haloperidol-sensitized Cebus monkeys are similar to those observed in humans with antipsychotic-induced dyskinesias (Marsden, 1985). When antipsychotic drug treatment is halted in humans exhibiting EPS, dyskinetic reactions frequently subside, but it is common for the dyskinetic reactions to return with the resumption of treatment. The return of dyskinesias following the resumption of treatment is considerably more rapid than that observed during the initial treatment. It is this rapid return of dyskinetic reactions produced by dyskinetic agents in humans that is the basis of our procedure in Cebus monkeys. At present, clozapine is the only antipsychotic agent for which cases of dyskinesias in humans are absent, and clozapine is the only antipsychotic agent tested that produces no dyskinetic reactions in the Cebus monkey, even when administered at maximally tolerated doses.

Migler et al (1993) exposed haloperidol-sensitized Cebus monkeys to a range of doses of haloperidol, thioridazine, clozapine, or quetiapine. The results are presented in Table 2. Haloperidol and thioridazine produced a high incidence of dyskinetic reactions. At oral doses of 0.25 to 1.0 mg/kg p.o., haloperidol produced dyskinetic reactions in all monkeys tested; thioridazine produced its maximum incidence of dyskinetic reactions (in 7 of 7 monkeys) at a dose of 5 mg/kg p.o..

TABLE 2. Dyskinetic Reactions in Sensitized Cebus Monkeys

Treatment	Dose (mg/kg p.o.)		Number of Monkeys With Dyskinetic Reactions/ Number Tested
Quetiapine	2.5		0/13
	5		1/13
	10		1/13
	20		2/13
	40		0/5
Clozapine	10		0/1
	20		0/13
	40		0/11
	60		0/5
Haloperidol	0.125		3/12
	0.250		6/6
	0.5		2/2
	1.0		13/13
Thioridazine	2.5		4/13
	5.0		7/7
	10.0		11/13

In contrast, quetiapine only produced dyskinetic reactions in 2 of 13 monkeys at 20 mg/kg p.o. and no dyskinetic reactions in 5 monkeys given 40 mg/kg p.o. The reactions that occurred with haloperidol or thioridazine were generally more intense than the reactions that occurred after quetiapine. Clozapine produced no dyskinetic reactions at any dose. Thus, the MED values (i.e., the lowest dose of drug producing dyskinetic responses in 50% of more of the monkeys tested) was 0.25 and 5 mg/kg p.o. for haloperidol and thioridazine, respectively. In marked contrast, a MED could not be established for quetiapine (i.e., it never produced more than a 15% incidence at any dose) and clozapine was totally inactive as an inducer of dyskinesia.

Goldstein and Snyder (1994) and Goldstein (1995) further evaluated the potential dyskinetic liability of quetiapine and other atypical antipsychotics in the haloperidol-sensitized monkey. They compared the dose range over which dyskinetic reactions occurred to the predicted antipsychotic dose range in monkeys based on clinical data. The results of this analysis are presented in Table 3.

TABLE 3. Dyskinetic Doses vs. Antipsychotic Doses for Quetiapine and Reference Agents in Haloperidol-Sensitized Cebus Monkeys

	Dose producing 100% incidence dyskinetic reactions (mg/kg PO)	Predicted antipsychotic dose range (mg/kg PO)
Quetiapine	>40	3-9
Clozapine	>60	6-18
Haloperidol	0.25	0.1-1
Olanzapine	0.5	0.2-0.6
Risperidone	0.125	0.08-0.16
Sertindole	2.5	0.24-0.48
Ziprasidone	0.62	0.8-3.2

Neither quetiapine nor clozapine produced significant (i.e., greater than 50%) incidence of dyskinetic reactions at doses well above the predicted antipsychotic dose range. Haloperidol produced a 100% incidence of dyskinetic reactions at the lower end of its predicted antipsychotic dose range. Risperidone and the other 'atypical' antipsychotics olanzapine and ziprasidone also produced 100% dyskinetic reactions at doses within the predicted antipsychotic dose range. Sertindole, while producing a 100% incidence of dyskinetic reactions, did so only at doses that exceeded the predicted antipsychotic dose range.

Inasmuch as the dyskinetic reactions in haloperidol-sensitized Cebus monkeys resemble EPS observed in humans after treatment with standard agents like haloperidol (Casey, 1995), these results suggest that quetiapine should have a reduced potential to cause EPS across the predicted antipsychotic dose range.

2.2 EFFECT OF QUETIAPINE AND SELECTED REFERENCE ANTIPSYCHOTICS IN DRUG-NAIVE CEBUS MONKEYS

Because quetiapine produced dyskinetic reactions in only a few haloperidol sensitized Cebus monkeys (see section 2.1), and those reactions were relatively weak in intensity, it appeared that it would have a reduced potential to produce antipsychotic-induced dyskinesias in humans. To confirm that suggestion, an additional paradigm was examined, specifically the ability to sensitize drug naive Cebus monkeys with quetiapine itself.

The preselected dose of 20 mg/kg p.o. of quetiapine was chosen by Migler et al (1993) for these studies because this dose had been previously shown to be sedating. Similarly, a dose of 20 mg/kg p.o. was selected for the clozapine group of monkeys since deaths had occurred at higher doses (40 mg/kg pp.o.) in sensitized Cebus monkeys. Although the 20 mg/kg pp.o. dose of clozapine produced no acute dystonic reactions, three of six monkeys died within the first five weeks of treatment. Consequently, the dose was reduced to a less sedating dose (10 mg/kg PO) and administered to the remaining 3 monkeys for the duration of the study (i.e., for an additional 7 weeks), and an additional monkey was included and dosed for 12 consecutive weeks. None of those four monkeys treated with clozapine exhibited acute dystonic reactions.

After 12 doses of haloperidol, 24 of 26 monkeys (92.3%) exhibited significant dyskinetic reactions. In contrast, after 12 doses of quetiapine, only seven of 13 (53.8%) exhibited dyskinetic reactions. Of the seven monkeys that exhibited dyskinetic reactions after treatment with quetiapine, three had weak reactions and did not react after being challenged for an additional 2 weeks. Thus, these three monkeys cannot be considered truly sensitized. No haloperidol-treated monkey ever failed to respond for 2 consecutive weeks after an initial dyskinetic reaction was observed. Haloperidol clearly produced more rapid sensitization, more intense reactions, and reactions of longer duration than was produced with quetiapine.

In order to compare the rate of sensitization of quetiapine and haloperidol in drug-naive Cebus monkeys, the cumulative percentage of monkeys exhibiting dyskinetic responses for the two treatment groups is plotted as a function of the number of weeks of treatment (Figure 2). Clearly, the haloperidol-treated monkeys exhibited a more rapid rate of sensitization, and a much higher percentage of monkeys (92.3%) were sensitized in the haloperidol group compared with the number sensitized in the quetiapine-treated groups (53.9% at the end of 12 weeks of treatment. Furthermore, since three of the seven monkeys treated with quetiapine responded weakly and then never responded again, it is questionable whether they should be considered sensitized. By excluding these 3 monkeys from the results presented in Figure 2 (as indicated by the dotted line), the cumulative percentage responding at the end of the study would be only 30.8% (four of 13).

Figure 2. A Comparison of the Rate of Sensitization of Quietiapine and Haloperidol in Drug-Naive Cebus Monkeys

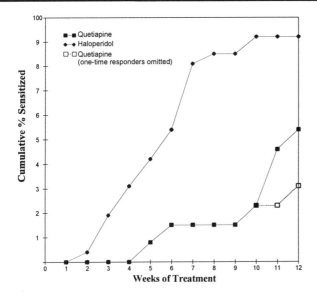

✱n = 13 for quietiapine and n=26 for haloperidol

Figure 3 presents the mean intensity rating for the quetiapine and haloperidol-treated groups as a function of the weeks of treatment. Because treatment was discontinued 2 weeks after the initial dyskinetic reaction occurred, the maximum intensity rating observed prior to discontinuation was used to represent the intensity of reaction for that monkey for the balance of the 12 weeks. It is evident from this figure that the initial reactions with haloperidol were observed as early as 2 weeks into the study, and their intensity rapidly increased over the course of the 12-week study. In marked contrast, the first weak response in the quetiapine-treated group was observed during week 5, and the intensity of the responses remained low throughout the study. Thus, haloperidol exhibited a steep intensity curve, whereas quetiapine exhibited an extremely shallow intensity curve.

FIGURE 3. A Comparison of Cumulative Weekly Dystonic Intensity Scores for Quetiapine and Haloperidol in Drug-Naive Cebus Monkeys*

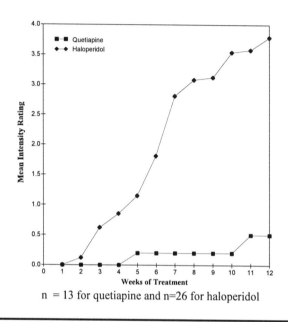

n = 13 for quetiapine and n=26 for haloperidol

The results obtained in drug-naive Cebus monkeys support the conclusion drawn from the studies performed in haloperidol-sensitized Cebus monkeys (see section 2.1). Specifically, quetiapine appears to have a markedly reduced potential to produce dyskinesias compared with haloperidol. Furthermore, the limited number of dyskinetic reactions that might occur exhibited a slower rate of onset and a markedly reduced intensity compared to haloperidol. Thus, the propensity for quetiapine to produce TD with chronic administration to humans is markedly less than that of typical antipsychotic agents.

2.3 EFFECT OF QUETIAPINE ON CATALEPSY IN RATS

Catalepsy is the most commonly used test in rodents to predict the potential liability of antipsychotics to produce EPS. An exception to this finding is clozapine, which does not produce EPS in humans yet produces some degree of catalepsy in the model (Migler et al., 1993). Comparing effective cataleptic doses with effective antipsychotic doses, as measured by the antagonism of DA agonist-mediated behaviors or elevation of DA metabolites, is another measure of EPS liability. In this paradigm, for example, there is a wider separation of doses with clozapine than with haloperidol.

Quetiapine and clozapine produced weak but statistically significant catalepsy at 20-40 mg/kg i.p.. However, at the highest dose tested (80 mg/kg i.p.) quetiapine, but not clozapine, produced a cataleptic effect equal to that of the highest dose of haloperidol tested (4 mg/kg i.p.). In view of the relatively high dose of quetiapine (80 mg/kg i.p.) required to produce haloperidol-like catalepsy compared to the lower doses (5-20 mg/kg i.p.) required to antagonize other DA agonist mediated behaviors, e.g., amphetamine-induced disruption of swimming or elevation of the DA metabolites DOPAC and HVA in rodents (see section 4.2), the EPS liability of quetiapine is more similar to clozapine than haloperidol.

3 EVALUATION OF QUETIAPINE IN ELECTROPHYSIOLOGIC STUDIES

3.1 REVERSAL OF D-AMPHETAMINE

The ability of a drug to reverse the inhibitory effect of D-amphetamine on DA cell firing in the motor-related substantia nigra zona compacta (A9) and limbic-related ventral tegmental (A10) areas has been used as a model to predict potential antipsychotic activity (Bunney, 1979; Bunney and Aghajanian, 1975; Bunney et al., 1973). All drugs with known antipsychotic properties have been shown to block and/or reverse the inhibitory effect of dopamine agonists on A9 and A10 DA cells (Bunney, 1979; Bunney and Aghajanian, 1975; Bunney et al., 1973). Drugs lacking antipsychotic properties (e.g., the phenothiazine analogs, promethazine and diethazine) were found to be without effect on DA systems (Bunney and Aghajanian, 1975; Bunney et al., 1973).

Quetiapine, over the dose range tested (0.5–4 mg/kgi.v.), significantly reversed the inhibitory effects of d-amphetamine on both A9 and A10 DA cells. Based on the ED50 for D-amphetamine reversal, quetiapine was almost three times more potent in the A10 area as compared to the A9 area (ED50s= 0.95 and 2.63 mg/kg i.v., respectively. Clozapine and thioridazine reversed the inhibitory effects of D-amphetamine on A9 and A10 DA cells at approximately the same doses. Haloperidol was the most potent antagonist tested, and reversed the inhibitory effects of d-amphetamine at 10 times lower doses in the A9 as compared to the A10 DA cells (ED50s= 0.007 and 0.074 mg/kg IV, respectively).

3.2 DOPAMINE CELL POPULATION STUDIES

Repeated 21–28 day oral administration of typical antipsychotic drugs (e.g. haloperidol, chlorpromazine) caused a decrease in the number of spontaneously active DA cells in both the A9 and A10 cell areas (White and Wang, 1983 Chiodo and Bunney, 1983). Glutamic acid, which normally depolarizes cell and causes them to fire, failed to activate these cells, whereas gamma aminobutyric acid (GABA), which normally hyperpolarizes cells and cause them to stop firing, paradoxically induced these cells to fire. It was proposed by White and Wang (1983) and Chiodo and Bunney (1983) that the inactivity o DA cells after chronic antipsychotic drug administration is due to the development of a state of tonic depolarization (depolarization inactivation) Therefore, an agent that repolarizes the cell through hyperpolarization (e.g. GABA, low-dose apomorphine) will restore spontaneous firing.

The development of depolarization inactivation of A10 DA cells was observed after the chronic administration of all antipsychotic drugs tested (White and Wang, 1983; Chiodo and Bunney, 1983). However, clozapine, an antipsychotic drug with a reduced propensity to induce neurological side effects, failed to cause depolarization inactivation of A9 DA cells. Therefore, the time-dependent inactivation of limbic-related A10 DA cells might be related to the antipsychotic efficacy of antipsychotic drugs, whereas the inactivation of motor-related A9 DA cell may be correlated with their side-effect liability.

Because it has also been reported (White and Wang, 1983; Chiodo and Bunney 1983) that single acute injections of antipsychotic drugs increased the number o spontaneously active DA cells only in the areas that were decreased by repeated treatment, these short-term acute effects could be used to predict both the therapeutic efficacy and side-effect liability of potential antipsychotic drugs These observations provided the rationale for determining the acute effects o quetiapine on the spontaneous activity of A9 and A10 DA cells. In addition, the profile of activity of quetiapine was compared to the reference antipsychotic drugs clozapine and haloperidol that were also tested under similar condition (Goldstein et al., 1993).

The acute effects of quetiapine, clozapine and haloperidol on the number o spontaneously active A9 and A10 cells are presented in the top panel of Figur 4. Quetiapine produced a dose-related increase in the number of active A10 DA cells. On A9 cells, the highest dose producing a significant increase in th number of active A10 DA cells (20 mg/kg p.o.) did not produce a significan increase in the number of active A9 DA cells. Thus, quetiapine had a selectiv effect on A10 DA cells. Clozapine exhibited a profile of activity (i.e., selectiv ncreases in the A10 area) that was very similar to quetiapine in terms of doses that produced equivalent effects and the magnitude of those effects. In contrast o the profile of activity exhibited by quetiapine and clozapine, haloperidol produced significant increases in the number of spontaneously active A9 and A10 DA cells at equivalent doses. Thus, the actions of haloperidol were not selective for either the A10 or A9 area.

The results of the chronic studies are shown in the bottom panel of Figure 4. Chronic administration of quetiapine produced a significant decrease in the number of spontaneously active DA cells only in the DA cell region in which he acute administration of quetiapine causes a significant increase in the number of active DA cells (i.e., A10 area). This decrease was significantly reversed by subsequent injection of a low dose of apomorphine, implying that the decrease was due to depolarization inactivation of the DA cells. A very similar profile of activity was observed after chronic administration of clozapine. In contrast, haloperidol caused a significant decrease in the number of active DA cells in both the A9 and A10 areas, an effect also reversed by njection of apomorphine suggesting depolarization inactivation had occurred.

The results of the electrophysiological studies presented in sections 3.1 and 3.2 clearly show that quetiapine has a profile of activity similar to that of clozapine. Quetiapine was active in tests predictive of antipsychotic activity (i.e., reversal of D-amphetamine and depolarization inactivation of A10 DA cells) but was relatively inactive in tests thought predictive of EPS (i.e., depolarization nactivation of A9 DA cells). Based on these studies, quetiapine is predicted to have antipsychotic properties with minimal EPS liability like clozapine.

4 EVALUATION OF QUETIAPINE IN NEUROCHEMICAL STUDIES

The neurochemical effects of quetiapine, particularly those on dopaminergic transmission, were evaluated in the following ways: (1) the affinity of quetiapine for DA and other neurotransmitter receptors was measured in vitro receptor binding studies; (2) the effects of quetiapine administration on DA metabolism were examined by measuring DA metabolite concentrations; (3) plasma prolactin concentrations, which are in part regulated by a tonic dopaminergic input, were also measured; (4) the in vivo occupancy of D_2 and 5-HT_2 receptors was estimated by measuring the ability of quetiapine to prevent receptor inactivation by N-ethoxycarbonyl-1, 2-dihydroquinoline (EEDQ); and (5) the effects of repeated administration of quetiapine on DA receptors was determined. In each of these investigations, quetiapine was compared with the atypical antipsychotic drug, clozapine.

4.1 IN VITRO STUDIES—RECEPTOR BINDING PROFILE

The ability of a drug to displace ligands that bind with a relatively high affinity and selectivity to a particular receptor provides a measure of the affinity of the drug for the specific receptor. The concentrations of quetiapine and clozapine that cause a 50% displacement (i.e., the IC_{50}) of specific receptor binding of various ligands are presented in Table 4. Quetiapine has low-to-moderate affinity at the DA D_1 and D_2 receptors ($IC_{50}s=1268$ nM and 329 nM, respectively), low-to-moderate affinity at serotonin 5-HT1A and 5-HT2 receptors (IC_{50} s=717nM and 148 nM, respectively), moderate to high affinity at $\alpha2$ and $\alpha1$ adrenergic receptors (IC_{50} s=271 nM and 94 nM, respectively), and no appreciable affinity at the muscarinic cholinergic or benzodiazepine receptors (IC_{50} s> 5000 nM).

Figure 4. Effects of Acute and Chronic 28-day Treatment with Quetiapine, Clozapine, Haloperidol or Vehicle on the Number of Spontaneously Active A9 and A10 Cells

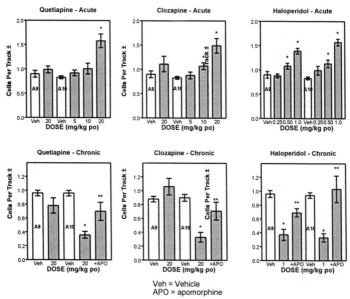

Veh = Vehicle
APO = apomorphine

* Significantly different from vehicle control value (Student's t-test, p<0.05)
** Significantly different from drug group (Student's t-test, p<0.05)

The receptor profile of quetiapine is similar to clozapine with respect to its interactions with a broad range of neurotransmitter receptors, and its low D_2 receptor affinity and higher receptor affinity 5-HT2. The latter property is considered predictive of an atypical antipsychotic agent (Meltzer, 1992). However, quetiapine also differs in its receptor profile from clozapine in not having appreciable affinity at the muscarinic cholinergic receptor ($IC_{50} > 10000$ nM). These findings predict that quetiapine should have fewer anticholinergic side effects, such as dry mouth, blurred vision, constipation, and difficulty passing urine, compared to clozapine.

Table 4. Affinities of Quietiapine and Clozapine for Various Receptors in Brain

Receptor	Ligand*	Quetiapine	Clozapine
		(IC_{50}#, nM)	
D_2	^{3}H-Spiperone	329	132
D_1	^{3}H-SCH 23390	1268	322
5-HT2	^{3}H-Ketanserin	148	20
5-HT1A	^{3}H-8-OH DPAT	717	316
$\alpha 1$	^{3}H Prazosin	94	50
$\alpha 2$	^{3}H-Rauwolscine	271	28
Muscarinic	^{3}H-QNB	>10000	287
Benzodiazepine	^{3}H-Flunitrazepam	>5000	>5000

* Per ligand, references to receptor-binding method used, respectively: Fields et al., 1977; Billard et al., 1984; Leysen et al., 1982; Hall et al., 1985; Greengrass and Bremner, 1979; Howe and Yakish, 1986; Yamamura and Snyder, 1974; Meiners and Salama, 1982.

Studies using a minimum of five concentrations of each drug in triplicate were used to determined IC50 values.

Additional receptor data on quetiapine were obtained through work performed at PanLabs Inc. PanLabs provided the opportunity to extend the profile of receptor binding for quetiapine by studying a much broader series of receptors than could be evaluated at Zeneca Pharmaceuticals. In addition to confirming the known receptor affinities of quetiapine at the DA D_1 and D_2, serotonin 5-HT$_2$ and 5-HT$_{1A}$, adrenergic α_1 and α_2 receptors, quetiapine was also found to have high affinity for both the histamine H$_1$ (IC_{50}=30 nM) and sigma (IC_{50}=90 nM) receptors. It is likely that the high affinity at the histamine H_1 receptor is a factor in the pharmacology of quetiapine and it may be related to the sedative properties of quetiapine. The evaluation of quetiapine in isolated tissues has also revealed potent H_1 antagonist properties (pK_B=9.4). The high affinity for quetiapine for the sigma receptor and the relevance of this property to the predicted therapeutic effects of quetiapine are not well understood.

Pan Labs also provided comparative binding data on cloned (human recombinant) dopamine D_1, D_2, D_3 and D_4 receptors (Table 5). Both quetiapine and clozapine (included as a reference agent) were initially evaluated at 10 μM. When inhibition above 50% occurred, it was followed up by IC_{50} determinations. Quetiapine demonstrated activity vs. D_1, D_2, and D_3 receptors, with descending receptor affinities (K_i nM, 293, 358, 469, respectively). Quetiapine had no appreciable affinity for the D_4 receptor (K_i > 10000 nM). Clozapine had a different profile on cloned dopamine receptors, exhibiting about equal affinity for the D_1 and D_4 receptor (K_i nM, 73,59, respectively) and lower affinity for the D_2 and D_3 receptors (K_i nM, 274, 449, respectively). High DA D_4 receptor affinity has been hypothesized to be a property which defines an atypical, i.e., clozapine-like, antipsychotic agent (Seeman, 1992). However, the relevance of D_4 receptor affinity and the distinction between typical and atypical antipsychotics has recently been challenged (Roth et al., 1995). Moreover, a recent clinical study by Kramer et al (1966) in which the effects of a selective D4 receptor antagonist (L-745,870) was evaluated in a chort of acutely psychotic schizophrenia patients, showed that L-745,870 caused an apparent worsening of psychosis relative to placebo. The authors' concluded that D_4 receptor antagonism is not associated with antipsychotic effects in humans.

Table 5. Cloned (human recombinant) Dopamine Receptor Binding (K_inM) for Quetiapine and Clozapine

Drug	D_1	D_2	D_3	D_4
Quetiapine	293	358	469	>10000
Clozapine	73	274	449	59

The human form of the serotonin 5-HT6 receptor has also recently been cloned, and affinity at this receptor has been linked to atypical antipsychotic, i.e., clozapine-like, actions (Roth et al., 1994). Quetiapine, like clozapine, was found to exhibit a high affinity for this receptor (K_i=33 and 9.5 nM, respectively) (Kohen et al., 1995). Thus, the 5-HT6 receptor affinity exhibited by quetiapine is consistent with an antipsychotic agent with predicted low EPS liability (Kohen et al., 1995).

Across a broad range of endogenous and cloned receptors, quetiapine exhibits binding properties that are similar to clozapine. Quetiapine has a relatively higher 5-HT$_2$ and 5-HT$_6$ receptor affinity relative to its DA D$_2$ receptor affinity, as well as having moderate-to-high affinity for the α_1 and α_2 adrenergic receptors, and H$_1$ histaminergic receptors. However, unlike clozapine, quetiapine lacks an appreciable affinity for the M$_1$ muscarinic cholinergic receptor, which may translate into it having fewer anticholinergic side effects relative to clozapine. Lack of affinity at the cloned DA D$_4$ receptor is another difference between quetiapine and clozapine, although the relevance of binding at the D$_4$ receptor to the atypical properties of clozapine remains unanswered. Quetiapine also demonstrates a high affinity for the sigma receptor, but the relevance of this receptor property to the known pharmacologic properties of antipsychotic drugs remains speculative.

4.2 IN VIVO STUDIES

(a) Effects on Dopamine (DA) Metabolism

The acute blockade of DA receptors results in a compensatory increase in brain levels of the DA metabolites DOPAC and HVA (Saller and Salama 1984, 1986a. This increase in DA metabolite levels provides an in vivo measure of a functional response to a DA receptor blockade, and the effects of quetiapine and clozapine were compared in this test.

Saller and Salama (1993) reported that 1 hour after oral administration, both quetiapine (20 mg/kg) and clozapine (20 mg/kg) produced similar statistically significant increases in DOPAC and HVA levels in the striatum, although quetiapine appeared more potent when administered intraperitoneally. These drugs also produced significant but smaller increases in HVA concentrations in the olfactory tubercle. Neither drug changed DOPAC concentrations in the olfactory tubercle.

The time course of the effects of quetiapine and clozapine on striatal DA turnover was also similar, peaking by 1 hour after both oral and intraperitoneal administration (Saller and Salama, 1993). Thus, based on these neurochemical measurements, the mode of action of quetiapine and clozapine appear similar, and the potency and duration of action of quetiapine would be at least equivalent to that of clozapine.

(b) Effects on Plasma Prolactin Concentrations

The most important endocrinological side effect of antipsychotic treatment in both laboratory animals and humans is a substantial increase in prolactin (PRL) secretion (Meltzer, 1992). In humans, this increase in PRL can lead to amenorrhea and galactorrhea (Meltzer, 1992). PRL secretion is under the direct inhibitory control of the tuberoinfindibular DA fibres and DA, via the stimulation of D_2 receptors and appears to tonically inhibit PRL secretion (Clemens et al., 1980; Saller and Salama, 1986b). It is not surprising that because of their DA D_2 antagonist action, all antipsychotics increase PRL after acute administration. However, the profile of clozapine in humans is different from that of other antipsychotics, in that it produces little or no PRL stimulation (Meltzer, 1992) and relatively brief changes in serum PRL.

The effects of acute administration of quetiapine on plasma PRL concentrations were therefore determined in rats for purposes of comparison to clozapine and haloperidol (Saller and Salama, 1993). The time course for the elevation in plasma PRL concentrations produced by the i.p. administration of quetiapine (20 mg/kg) compared with clozapine (20 mg/kg), haloperidol (0.25 mg/kg) and vehicle (HPMC) is presented in Figure 5; and, the time course for the elevation in plasma PRL concentrations produced by the p.o.administration of quetiapine (20 mg/kg) compared to clozapine (20 mg/kg) and vehicle (HPMC) is shown in Figure 6.

A small increase in plasma PRL concentrations was observed after vehicle (HPMC) administration in both the i.p. and p.o.studies, and is probably due to the stress associated with the steps of injection. Quetiapine and haloperidol increased plasma PRL concentrations after i.p. administration. The magnitude of the increase was greater with quetiapine compared to haloperidol. However, the time course for these effects differed. In the quetiapine-treated rats, the increase in plasma PRL concentrations following both i.p.(Figure 5) and p.o. (Figure 6) administration peaked at 15 minutes and returned toward control values by 120 minutes, although the levels were still significantly increased compared to the control value for this time point. In contrast, PRL concentrations remained elevated over time after the i.p. administration of haloperidol (Figure 5). In clozapine-treated rats, there was a small and variable change in plasma PRL concentrations, increasing slightly after i.p. administration (Figure 5), and decreasing slightly after p.o. administration (Figure 6).

Thus, quetiapine produced elevations in plasma PRL concentrations that declined rapidly over time, which is consistent with the profile of an atypical antipsychotic agent.

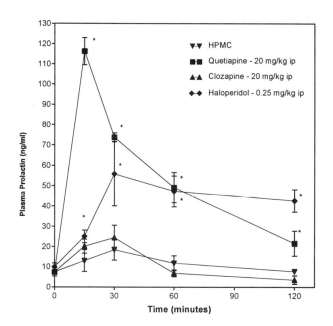

Significantly different from control, p<0.05 (Student's two tailed t-test). n = 6 to 8 rats per treatment group.

Figure 5   Effect of Intraperitoneal Quietiapine, Clozapine, or Haloperidol on Plasma Prolactin Levels

(c) DA and 5-HT2 Receptor Occupancy

The occupancy of D_2 and 5-HT_2 receptors by quetiapine and clozapine was estimated by measuring the ability of these drugs to prevent receptor inactivation by n-ethoxycarbonyl-1,2-dihydroquinoline (EEDQ). Both quetiapine and clozapine provided significantly greater protection of 5-HT_2 than D_2 receptors. Likewise, the D_2 receptor occupancy by either drug appeared to decline more rapidly than the occupancy of 5-HT_2 receptors. For the purpose of comparisons, the receptor occupancy produced by haloperidol was also determined. Haloperidol afforded a high level of protection at D_2 sites that was maintained throughout the 4-hour test period. No detectable protection was afforded to the 5-HT$_2$ sites by haloperidol.

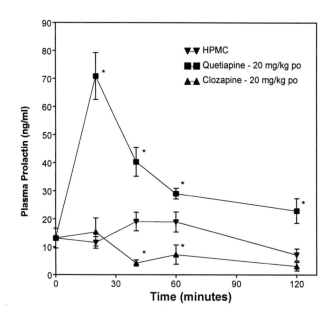

Figure 6. Effect of Oral Quetiapine or Clozapine on Plasma Prolactin Levels

The results of these studies showed that quetiapine exhibited greater receptor occupancy at the 5-HT$_2$ compared with the D_2 receptor, which is a profile shared by clozapine but not by haloperidol. Having greater 5-HT$_2$ relative to D_2 occupancy is a feature of an atypical antipsychotic drug that may be related to a lower propensity to cause EPS (Meltzer, 1992).

4.3 EFFECT OF REPEATED ADMINISTRATION OF QUETIAPINE ON DA RECEPTORS

Numerous studies have shown that chronic administration of typical antipsychotics will result in D_2 receptor supersensitivity in the striatal region of the brain (Seeman, 1980). Using receptor binding studies, this is taken as evidence of an increase in the number (B_{max}) of D_2 receptors (Seeman, 1980). Moreover, it has been suggested that the development of DA receptor supersensitivity in the striatum may be related to the occurrence of TD (Klawans, 1973), although the relationship is controversial. Clozapine, which is characterized by its nondyskinetic liability, has not generally been reported to increase the number of DA receptors in rats after repeated administration (Klawans, 1973). The chronic administration of quetiapine or clozapine (20 mg/kg IP) did not increase the number of striatal D_2 receptors (Table 6). To the extent that lack of D_2 receptor supersensitivity at drug dosages which appear to block DA receptors is indicative of TD, these data point to a low propensity for quetiapine to produce TD.

Table 6. The Effect of Repeated Administration of Either Quetiapine or Clozapine on ^{3}H-spiroperidol binding to rat striatal membranes.

Treatment	KD ± SEM			Bmax ± SEM		
		(n M)			(fmol/mg tissue)	
Control	0.3 2	±	0.0 6	30.6	±	4.3
Quetiapine (20 mg/kg IP)	0.4 0	±	0.1 0	35.8	±	5.1
Control	0.2 9	±	0.0 3	65.6	±	3.1
Clozapine (20 mg/kg IP)	0.3 1	±	0.0 7	59.8	±	8.6

* N = 16 rats per treatment group.

5 FURTHER STUDIES DEMONSTRATING A CLOZAPIINE-LIKE PROFILE FOR QUETIAPINE

5.1 EARLY GENE EXPRESSION

Clozapine and haloperidol produce different induction patterns of c-fos expression in the forebrain. Haloperidol increases fos-like immunoreactivity (FLI) in both the motor-related (i.e., dorsolateral striatum) and limbic-related (i.e., nucleus accumbens, lateral septum, and prefrontal cortical) areas, while clozapine produces such effects only in the limbic-related areas (Robertson et al., 1994). Accordingly, it was deemed possible with this approach to characterize the EPS liability of antipsychotic agents. A range of standard antipsychotics with documented liability for producing EPS, like chlorpromazine, fluphenazine, haloperidol, loxapine, metoclopramide, and molindone, as well as atypical agents such as clozapine, quetiapine, risperidone, fluperlapine, and others, were examined for their effects on the regional expression of FLI (Robertson et al., 1994).

Consistent with the hypothesis that FLI is elevated in the dorsolateral striatum by antipsychotic drugs having EPS liability, all the standard agents elevated expression of FLI in this structure. In addition, all the standard agents elevated FLI in the nucleus accumbens and medial striatum, indicating that potential antipsychotic activity may be associated with this site. In contrast, compounds less likely to produce EPS such as clozapine, quetiapine, fluperlapine, risperidone, and others either failed to increase or produced minor elevations in FLI in the dorsolateral striatum (Robertson et al., 1994).

The results of these studies suggest that there is a strong correlation between the ability of a compound to increase FLI in the dorsolateral striatum and its liability for producing EPS. Quetiapine was like clozapine in this regard and failed to elevate FLI in this structure. Inasmuch as the EPS liability of an antipsychotic agent is correlated with induction of FLI in the dorsolateral striatum, quetiapine is predicted to be clozapine-like and have minimal EPS liability.

5.2 DRUG DISCRIMINATION IN SQUIRREL MONKEYS

Squirrel monkeys can be trained to discriminate between clozapine and saline injections by differentially responding on the left or right lever in an operant box, depending on whether clozapine (1 mg/kg) or saline was injected. Once trained, the monkeys can be used to reliably detect the presence of a clozapine-like drug by their choice of the appropriate lever (Carey and Bergman, 1994).

In clozapine-trained monkeys, quetiapine, perlapine, and several experimental dibenzazepines produced dose-dependent increases in drug-appropriate responding with full substitution for clozapine at the highest doses (Carey and Bergman, 1994). In contrast, remoxipride, clothiapine, and loxapine did not produce drug-appropriate responding. In addition, risperidone failed to substitute for clozapine in any of the monkeys studied (Carey and Bergman, 1994). Although the nature of the stimulus detected by the monkeys is unknown, the results suggest that the monkeys sense the same clozapine-like stimulus properties when injected with quetiapine.

5.3 JAVA MONKEY SOCIAL ISOLATION

There is evidence showing that antipsychotic drugs, with the notable exception of clozapine, are not very effective in reversing negative symptoms. The search for a clozapine-like drug has been hampered by the lack of a good animal model for negative symptoms. However, one of the few aspects of negative symptoms that can be measured in animals is social withdrawal (Ellenbroek, 1991; Ellenbroek et al., 1991). This effect can be induced in monkeys treated with amphetamine. Data suggest that the effects of amphetamine on social behavior in monkeys represents an animal model with a certain degree of predictive validity for the negative symptoms of schizophrenia. This is further emphasized by the finding that standard antipsychotics do not affect this social isolation (Schiorring, 1977; Miczek and Yoshimura, 1982)

Quetiapine in different doses was able to reverse most of the effects of amphetamine in Java monkeys (Ellenbroek et al., 1996). These included a reversal of the amphetamine-induced decrease in social behavior as measured by increases in passive grooming and increases in active and passive proximity. In addition, quetiapine reduced the amphetamine-induced increase in the frequency of active submissive behavior. This latter behavior has been suggested to be a model for paranoid delusions (Ellenbroek, 1991).

Inasmuch as the amphetamine-induced social isolation model in Java monkeys represents an animal model for the positive and negative symptoms of schizophrenia, quetiapine is predicted to have clinical efficacy in these aspects of the illness.

5.4 PAW TEST

The paw test measures the ability of a rat to spontaneously withdraw its forelimbs and hindlimbs (Ellenbroek et al., 1987). Using several different criteria, it can be shown that prolongation of the forelimb retraction time can be regarded as an animal model for EPS, whereas prolongation of the hindlimb retraction time can be regarded as an animal model for antipsychotic efficacy. Thus the paw test is able to differentiate between classical antipsychotic drugs (which increase both the forelimb and hindlimb retraction times) and atypical antipsychotic drugs (which increase only the hindlimb retraction time) (Ellenbroek et al., 1987).

Quetiapine was evaluated in the paw test (Ellenbroek et al., 1996), and produced a dose-related increase in hindlimb retraction time. The minimal effective dose for producing a statistically significant effect was 25 mg/kg IP. In contrast, only at the highest dose tested (100 mg/kg IP) was there evidence of a statistically significant increase in forelimb retraction time. On the basis of this test, there appears to be a fourfold separation between doses that affect hindlimb retraction time (predictive of antipsychotic potential) and doses that affect forelimb retraction time. This ratio of four compares favorably with clozapine (ratio >5) and is disparate (predictive of EPS liability) from the classical antipsychotic agents, e.g., haloperidol and chlorpromazine (ratios=1), and further points toward quetiapine being a potential antipsychotic agent with low EPS liability.

5.5 PREPULSE INHIBITION TEST

Prepulse inhibition of the acoustic startle reflex has been used as an animal model with face validity for the sensorimotor gating deficits in schizophrenic patients (Swerdlow et al., 1990; Swerdlow and Geyer, 1992). In humans and rats, the startle reflex is inhibited when the startling stimulus is preceded by a weak prepulse, and this prepulse inhibition (PPI) is reduced or eliminated in schizophrenic patients and in rats pretreated with the dopamine agonist apomorphine. A range of antipsychotics, including clozapine, have been shown to restore PPI in apomorphine-treated rats, and their effects in this model strongly correlate with their clinical potency (Swerdlow et al., 1990; Swerdlow and Geyer, 1992).

Swerdlow and colleagues (Swerdlow et al., 1994) studied the ability of quetiapine to restore PPI in apomorphine-treated rats, comparing the results of quetiapine to clozapine. Both quetiapine and clozapine significantly restored PPI, with quetiapine being slightly more potent than clozapine. There was also a trend toward an increase in PPI induced by quetiapine, although the effects were not statistically significant. However, in this regard the magnitude of the increase in PPI at the threshold dose of quetiapine (5 mg/kg s.c.) is comparable to that produced by a high dose of clozapine (12 mg/kg s.c.) (Swerdlow and Geyer, 1992). Thus, quetiapine resembled clozapine in these tests by restoring PPI disrupted by apomorphine, and exhibited a trend toward enhancing sensorimotor gating in rats.

SUMMARY AND CONCLUSIONS

This review has focused on the pharmacologic properties of quetiapine that predict antipsychotic actions and minimal EPS liability. Quetiapine was shown to be active in classical tests for antipsychotic activity, such as conditioned avoidance in primates, with potency greater than clozapine in higher nonhuman species. It was also shown to reverse the actions of dopamine agonists measured either behaviorally or electrophysiologically in mice, rats, cats, and monkeys. Quetiapine was also shown to elevate levels of the dopamine metabolites HVA and DOPAC in brain, which are considered to be neurochemical indices of a dopamine D_2 receptor blockade, and produces a transient elevation in plasma prolactin levels after acute administration in rats. Quetiapine also reversed amphetamine-induced disruption of social behavior in Java monkeys, which is similar to clozapine but unlike haloperidol. Inasmuch as this model mimics the negative symptoms of schizophrenia, quetiapine is predicted to have efficacy in this component of the disease. Full substitution for clozapine in a monkey drug discrimination paradigm provides further evidence for clozapine-like actions.

In tests predictive of EPS, quetiapine was found to be unlike standard antipsychotics and to have the following profile: a low affinity for the DA D_2 receptor and a higher $5\text{-}HT_2$ relative to D_2 receptor-binding ratio, a profile further confirmed in in vivo receptor occupancy studies; it does not produce dopamine D_2 receptor supersensitivity after chronic administration; produce only weak catalepsy at effective dopamine D_2 receptor-blocking doses; selectivity for the limbic system by producing depolarization blockade of the A10 mesolimbic but not the A9 nigrostriatal dopamine-containing neurons following the chronic administration of drug and increases c-fos expression in limbic- but not motor-related regions after acute and chronic administration. In addition, it exhibits minimal dystonic liability over the predicted antipsychotic dose-range in haloperidol-sensitized or drug-naive Cebus monkeys after acute and chronic administration. It has been hypothesized that agents with a low EPS liability may also have a low potential liability to produce tardive dyskinesia.

On the basis of the above preclinical findings, it would be predicted that quetiapine will have an atypical antipsychotic profile and be less likely to cause EPS in humans. In the next chapter, Dr. Lisa Arvanitis reviews the clinical findings with quetiapine. These findings will confirm the predicted preclinical profile and show that quetiapine is indeed an atypical antipsychotic drug.

REFERENCES

Billard, W., Ruperto, V., Crosby, G., Iorio, L.C. and Barnett, A. (1984) "Characterization of the binding of 3H–SCH 23390, a selective D1 receptor antagonist ligand, in rat striatum". Life Sci. 35, 1885–1893.

Bunney, B.S. (1979) "The electrophysiological pharmacology of midbrain dopaminergic systems". In: The Neurobiology of Dopamine (Eds. A.S. Horn, J. Korf, B.H.C. Westerink), Academic Press, New York, pp 417–452.

Bunney, B.S. and Aghajanian, G.K. (1975) "The effect of antipsychotic drugs on the firing of dopaminergic neurons: a reappraisal". In: Antipsychotic Drugs, Pharmacodynamics and Pharmacokinetics (Eds. G. Sedvall, B. Uvnas and Y. Zotterman), Pergamon, New York, pp 305–318.

Bunney, B.S., Walters, J.R., Roth, R.H. and Aghajanian, G.K. (1973) "Dopaminergic neurons: effect of antipsychotic drugs and amphetamine on single cell activity". J. Pharmacol. Exp. Ther. 185, 560–571.

Carey, G. and Bergman, J. (1994) "Discriminative stimulus effects of proposed atypical neuroleptics in clozapine–trained squirrel monkeys". Behav. Pharmacol. 5 (Suppl. 1), 114.

Casey, D.E. (1995) "Neuroleptic–induced acute extrapyramidal syndromes and tardive dyskinesia". In: Schizophrenia UK (Eds. S.R. Hirsch and D. R. Weinberger), Blackwell Science Ltd, London, pp 546–565.

Casey, D.E., Gerlach, J. and Christensson, E. (1980) "Dopamine, acetylcholine, and GABA effects in acute dystonia in primates". Psychopharmacology 70, 83–87.

Chiodo, L.A. and Bunney, B.S. (1983) "Typical and atypical neuroleptics: differential effects of chronic administration on the activity of A9 and A10 midbrain dopaminergic neurons". J. Neurosc. 3, 1607–1619.

Clemens, J.A., Shaar, C.J. and Smalstig, E.B. (1980) "Dopamine, PIF, and other regulators of prolactin secretion". Fed. Proc. 39, 2907–2911.

Ellenbroek, B.A. (1991) "The ethological analysis of monkeys in a social setting as an animal model for schizophrenia". In: Animal Models in Psychopharmacology (Eds. B. Olivier, J. Mos and J.L. Slangen), Birkhauser Verlag, Basel, pp 265–284.

Ellenbroek, B.A., Peeters, B.W., Honig, W.M. and Cools, A.R. (1987) "The paw test: a behavioral paradigm for differentiating between classical and atypical neuroleptic drugs". Psychopharmacology 93, 343–348.

Ellenbroek, B.A., Willemen, A.P.M. and Cools, A.R. (1991) "Are antagonists of the dopamine D_1 receptors drugs that attenuate both positive and negative symptoms of schizophrenia? A pilot study in Java monkeys". Neuropsychopharmacology 2, 191–199.

Ellenbroek, B.A., Lubbers, L.J. and Cools, A.R. (1996) "The activity of 'Seroquel' (ICI 204,636) in animal models for atypical properties of antipsychotics: a comparison with clozapine". Neuropsychopharmacology (in press).

Fields, J.Z., Reisine, T.D. and Yamamura, H.I. (1977) "Biochemical demonstration of dopaminergic receptors in rat and human brain using [^{3}H]spiroperidol". Brain Res. 136, 578–584.

Goldstein, J.M., Snyder, D.H. (1994) "Effects of SEROQUEL, clozapine and other atypical agents in primate models of EPS". Schizoph. Bull. 15:152.

Goldstein, J.M. (1995) "Preclinical tests that predict clozapine–like atypical antipsychotic actions". In:Critical Issues in the Treatment of Schizophrenia (Eds. N. Brunello, G. Racagni, S.Z. Langer, and J. Mendlewicz), Karger, Basel, pp 95–101.

Goldstein, J.M., Litwin, L.C., Sutton, E.J. and Malick, B.M. (1993) "Seroquel: electrophysiological profile of a potential atypical antipsychotic". Psychopharmacology 112, 293–298.

Greengrass, D. and Bremner, R. (1979) "Binding characteristics of ^{3}H–prazosin to rat brain α–adrenergic receptors". Eur. J. Pharmacol. 55, 323–326.

Gulmann, N.C., Bahr, B., Andersen, B. and Eliassen, H.M.M. (1976) "A double–blind trial of baclofen against placebo in the treatment of schizophrenia". Acta Psychiatr. Scand. 54, 287–293.

Hall, M.D., Mestikawy, S.E., Emerit, M.B., Pichat, L., Hamon, M. and Gozlan, H. (1985) "[^{3}H]8–hydroxy–2–(Di–n–propylamino) tetralin binding to pre– and postsynaptic 5–hydroxytryptamine sites in various regions of the rat brain". J. Neurochem. 44, 1685–1696.

Howe, J.R., Yaksh, T.L. (1986) Characterization of [^{3}H]rauwolscine binding to alpha$_2$– adrenoceptor sites in the lumbar spinal cord of the cat: comparison to such binding sites in the cat frontal cerebral cortex". Brain Res. 368, 87–100.

Karson, C., Freed, W.J., Kleinman, J.E., Bigelow, L.B. and Wyatt, R.J. (1981) "Neuroleptics decrease blinking in schizophrenic subjects". Biol. Psychiatry 16, 679– 682.

Klawans, H.L. (1973) "The pharmacology of tardive dyskinesias". Am. J. Psychiatry 130, 82–86.

Kohen, R., Mercalf, M.A., Kahn, N., Druck, T., Huebner, K., Lachowicz, J.E., Meltzer, H.Y., Sibley, D.R., Roth, B.L., and Hamblin, M.W. (1995) "Cloning, characterization, and chromosomal localization of a human 5–HT6 serotonin receptor". J. Neurochem. (in press)

Kramer, M.S., Zimbrosf, D., Last, B., Getson, A. and the D4 Antagonist Study Group (1996) "The effects of a selective D4 antagonist (L–745,870) in acutely psychotic schizophrrenic patients". Poster number 106 presentation at the 36th Annual Meeting of the New Clinical Drug Evaluation Unit, Boca Raton, FL, May 28–31.

Leysen, J.E., Niemegeers, G.J.E., Van Nueten, J.M. and Laduron, P.M. (1982) "[3H]Ketanserin (R 41 468), a selective 3H–ligand for serotonin2 receptor binding sites Binding properties, brain distribution, and functional role". Mol. Pharmacol. 21, 301–314.

Marsden, C.D. (1985) "Is tardive dyskinesia a unique disorder?" In: Dyskinesia – Research and Treatment (Eds. D.E. Casey, T. N. Chase, A. V. Christense, and J Gerlach), Springer–Verlag, Berlin, pp 64–71.

Meiners, B.M. and Salama, A.I. (1982) "Enhancement of benzodiazepine and GABA binding by the novel anxiolytic, tracazolate". Eur. J. Pharmacol. 78, 315–322.

Meltzer, H.Y. (1992) "The mechanism of action of clozapine in relation to its clinica advantages". In: Novel Antipsychotic Drugs (Ed. H.Y. Meltzer), Raven Press, New York, pp 1–13.

Meltzer, H.Y., Daniels, S. and Fang, V.S. (1975) "Clozapine increases rat serum prolactin levels". Life Sci. 17, 339–342.

Miczek, K. and Yoshimura, H. (1982) "Disruption of primate social behavior by D-amphetamine and cocaine: differential antagonism by antipsychotics" Psychopharmacology 76, 163–171.

Migler, B.M., Wawara, E.J. and Malick, J.B. (1993) "Seroquel: behavioral effects in conventional and novel tests for atypical antipsychotic drug". Psychopharmacology 112 299–307.

Robertson, G.S., Matsumura, H. and Fibiger, H.C. (1994) "Induction patterns of Fos–like immunoreactivity in the forebrain as predictors of atypical antipsychotic activity". J Pharmacol. Exp. Ther. 271, 1058–1066.

Roth, B.L., Craigo, S.C., Choudhary, M.S., Uluer, A., Monsma, F.J. Jr., Shen, Y. Meltzer, H.Y. and Sibley, D.R. (1994) "Binding of typical and atypical antipsychotic agents to 5–hydroxytryptamine–6 and 5–hydroxytryptamine–7 receptors". J. Pharmacol Exp. Ther. 268, 1403–1410.

Roth, B.L., Tandra, S., Burgess, L.H., Sibley, D.R. and Meltzer, H.Y. (1995) "D4 dopamine receptor binding affinity does not distinguish between typical and atypical antipsychotic drugs". Psychopharmacology 120, 365–368.

Saller, C.F. and Salama, A.I. (1984) "Rapid automated analysis of biogenic amines and their metabolites using reverse phase HPLC with electrochemical detection". J. Chromatogr. 309, 287–298.

Sller, C.F. and Salama, A.I. (1986a) "3–Methoxytyramine accumulation: effects of typical neuroleptics and various atypical compounds". Naunyn–Schmiedeberg's Arch. Pharmacol. 334, 125–132.

Saller, C.F. and Salama, A.I. (1986b) "D–1 dopamine receptor stimulation elevates plasma prolactin levels". Eur. J. Pharmacol. 122, 139–142.

Saller, C.F. and Salama, A.I. (1993) "Seroquel: biochemical profile of a potential atypical antipsychotic". Psychopharmacology 112, 285–292.

Saller, C.F., Kreamer, L.D., Adamovage, L.A. and Salama, A.I. (1989) "Dopamine receptor occupancy in vivo: measurement by using N–ethoxycarbonyl–1,2–dihydroquinoline (EEDQ)". Life Sci. 45, 917–929.

Schiorring, E. (1977) "Changes in individual and social behavior induced by amphetamine and related compounds in monkeys and man". In: Cocaine and Other Stimulants (Eds. E. Ellinwood and M. Kilbey), Plenum Press, New York, pp 481–522.

Seeman, P. (1980) "Brain dopamine receptors". Pharmacol. Rev. 32, 229–313.

Seeman, P. (1992) "Dopamine receptor sequences. Therapeutic levels of neuroleptics occupy D_2 receptors, clozapine occupies D_4". Neuropsychopharmacology 7, 261–284.

Simpson, G., Branchey, M.H. and Shrivastava, R.K. (1976) "Baclofen in schizophrenia". Lancet 1(Issue No 7966), 966–967.

Stevens, J.R. (1978) "Eye blink and schizophrenia: psychosis or tardive dyskinesia?" Am. J. Psychiatry 135, 223–226.

Swerdlow, N.R. and Geyer, M.A. (1992) "Clozapine and haloperidol in an animal model of sensorimotor gating deficits in schizophrenia". Pharmacol. Biochem. Behav. 44, 741–744.

Swerdlow, N.R., Keith, V.A., Braff, D.L., and Geyer, M.A. (1990) "Effects of spiperone, raclopride, SCH 23390 and clozapine on apomorphine inhibition of sensorimotor gating of the startle response in the rat". J. Pharmacol. Exp. Ther. 256, 530–536.

Swerdlow, N.R., Zisook, D. and Taaid, N. (1994) "Seroquel (ICI 204,636) restores prepulse inhibition of acoustic startle in apomorphine–treated rats: similarities to clozapine". Psychopharmacology 114, 675–678.

Weiss, B., Santelli, S., and Lusink, G. (1977) "Movement disorders induced in monkeys by chronic haloperidol treatment". Psychopharmacology 53, 283–293.

White, F.J. and Wang, R.Y. (1983) "Differential effects of classical and atypical antipsychotic drugs on A9 and A10 dopamine neurons". Science 221, 1054–1057.

Worms, P., Broekkamp, C.L.E., and Lloyd, K.G. (1983) "Behavioral effects of neuroleptics". In: Neuroleptics: Neurochemical Behavioral and Clinical Perspectives (Eds. J.T. Coyle and S. J. Enna), Raven Press, New York, pp 93–117.

Yamamura, H.I. and Snyder, S.H. (1974) "Muscarinic cholinergic binding in rat brain". Proc. Natl. Acad. Sci. (USA) 71, 1725–1729.

11

CLINICAL PROFILE OF SEROQUEL™ (QUETIAPINE): AN OVERVIEW OF RECENT CLINICAL STUDIES

Lisa A. Arvanitis

INTRODUCTION

Recent advances in schizophrenia research have provided new insight into the pathophysiology of this serious psychiatric disorder. Based on these understandings, pharmaceutical researchers have been able to selectively screen potential drug candidates for compounds with antipsychotic properties but without the liabilities associated with the older agents. Although the antipsychotic agents from the 1950s to 1980s provide substantial relief from the positive symptoms of schizophrenia (delusions and hallucinations), for as many as 70% to 80% of patients, the benefit is only partial (Hegarty et al., 1994). Some are simply resistant to treatment; others find relief from the delusions and hallucinations but are plagued by the core negative symptoms associated with schizophrenia (affective flattening, avolition, and social withdrawal). Still others fail to show long-term improvement. Even when these older antipsychotics have produced relatively good clinical benefit, many patients take their medications inconsistently or discontinue them altogether because of troubling adverse effects (e.g., extrapyramidal signs and symptoms [EPS], sexual dysfunction) or because of the cognitive impairments stemming from either the schizophrenia itself or the medications taken to control the symptoms. With the limitations in therapy, many patients become increasingly ill and have greater numbers of residual symptoms (both positive and negative) and exhibit a decline in their

Schizophrenia: Breaking Down the Barriers. Edited by S.G. Holliday, R.J. Ancill and G.W. MacEwan. © 1996 John Wiley & Sons Ltd

capacity to function (McGlashan, 1988). The challenge for researchers, therefore, is to find agents that will bring about a more substantial reduction of both the positive and negative symptoms as well as the cognitive dysfunction associated with schizophrenia and improve overall outcome, yet produce few adverse effects.

Seroquel™ (Quetiapine, Zeneca Pharmaceuticals) is one of a new class of "atypical" antipsychotics developed with the benefits of recent research. According to Meltzer and colleagues (Meltzer, 1991; Meltzer et al., 1989) and Casey (Casey, 1992), drugs are classifiable as atypical if any of the following criteria are met:

• Clinical trials indicate antipsychotic activity with minimal EPS.

• Clinical experience suggests no causation of tardive dyskinesia (TD) or elevation of serum prolactin.

• Preclinical studies demonstrate weak or no cataleptic potential.

In the preceding chapter, Dr. Jeffrey Goldstein reviewed the preclinical pharmacological studies with quetiapine that have highlighted its profile as an atypical antipsychotic agent. He presented data from a battery of preclinical tests that predicted quetiapine would have antipsychotic activity, efficacy for negative symptoms, low liability for EPS, and no sustained rise in plasma prolactin levels. On the basis of these positive findings in the preclinical studies, quetiapine was entered into an international clinical development program. This chapter will review the comparative studies of quetiapine's efficacy, safety, and tolerability in hospitalized patients with acute exacerbations of chronic or subchronic schizophrenia. These studies confirm the preclinical prediction that quetiapine would be a well-tolerated atypical antipsychotic with efficacy for both positive and negative symptoms with negligible EPS and without the induction of hyperprolactinemia. Ongoing animal pharmacology studies, which Dr. Goldstein also presented, continue to confirm the initial preclinical profile. A review of the results of the promising clinical studies follows, focusing on the multicenter trials involving comparisons with placebo or chlorpromazine conducted during Phase II clinical development.

1. EVIDENCE FOR THE EFFICACY, SAFETY, AND TOLERABILITY OF QUETIAPINE AS AN ATYPICAL ANTIPSYCHOTIC

1.1 OVERVIEW OF STUDIES

The efficacy, safety, and tolerability of quetiapine in the treatment of hospitalized patients with acute exacerbations of chronic or subchronic schizophrenia have been evaluated in four Phase II clinical studies, three of which were placebo-controlled trials, and one of which was an active control study. Study 4 was a single-center, rising dose, pharmacokinetic, tolerability and pilot efficacy study (Fabre et al., 1995). Studies 6 and 8 were larger, multicenter trials of the efficacy and tolerability of quetiapine. In Study 6, a 12-center study conducted in the United States, quetiapine, in doses up to 750 mg per day was compared to placebo (Borison et al., 1996). In Study 8, an international study involving 24 sites, high-dose (up to 750 mg/day) and low-dose (up to 250 mg/day) quetiapine were compared to placebo (Small et al., Submitted). The last of the Phase II multicenter studies, Study 7, was an active-controlled trial in which quetiapine (up to 750 mg/day) was compared to chlorpromazine (up to 750 mg/day) at 27 centers in Europe and South Africa (Peuskens and Link, Submitted).

An international Phase III clinical development program is underway. Two 6-week, multicenter, double-blind, controlled trials evaluating the efficacy, tolerability, and optimal dose range and dose regimen of quetiapine in the treatment of patients with acute exacerbations of schizophrenia have recently been completed. Study 13 was a North American placebo-controlled trial, which evaluated five fixed doses of quetiapine (75, 150, 300, 600, and 750 mg daily) and one fixed dose of haloperidol (12 mg daily) (Arvanitis and Miller, in preparation; Arvanitis, 1995). Study 12 was an international trial in which two dose regimens of quetiapine (450 mg daily, administered either in two or three times daily doses; and, 50 mg daily, administered in twice daily doses) were evaluated (King et al., In preparation). A number of additional Phase III studies are ongoing. These include: a North American, multicenter study in patients with treatment resistant schizophrenia; open-label extensions of completed trials to evaluate long-term safety and efficacy; and a study to assess the efficacy and safety of quetiapine in elderly patients with a variety of psychotic disorders. Other studies have been designed to evaluate particular pharmacokinetic and pharmacodynamic issues, including the use of quetiapine in special patient populations (i.e., renally or hepatically impaired), and the potential interactions from the concomitant use of quetiapine with CYP450 enzyme inducers (phenytoin) and inhibitors (cimetidine), or with frequently used central nervous system drugs (lithium and lorazepam). Two positron emission tomography

(PET) studies are underway in patients with schizophrenia to evaluate the dopamine D_2 and serotonin 5-HT_2 receptor occupancy of quetiapine. The first, designed to support once or twice daily dosing of quetiapine, is a study of the time course of D_2 and 5-HT_2 receptor occupancy opposite the time course of quetiapine plasma concentrations over a 24-hour period (Gefvert et al., 1995). The second is an evaluation of the relationship between the dose of quetiapine and the occupancy of D_2 and 5-HT_2 receptors across the therapeutic dose range.

1.2   PATIENTS AND METHODS

1.2.1   Demographics/Inclusion–Exclusion Criteria for Phase II Studies

With some minor exceptions, the patient populations evaluated consisted of hospitalized subjects aged 18 through 60 who met the criteria for acute exacerbations of chronic or subchronic schizophrenia according to the Diagnostic and Statistical Manual of Mental Disorders, 3rd Edition, Revised (DSM-III-R) (American Psychiatric Association, 1987). In order to be included in studies, patients were required to meet the following key criteria:

(1) A minimum total score on the 18-item Brief Psychiatric Rating Scale (Overall, 1962) of 45 (1-7 point scoring) or 27 (0-6 point scoring).

(2) At least a "moderate" rating on two of four of the individual BPRS positive-symptom cluster items—conceptual disorganization, suspiciousness, hallucinatory behavior, unusual thought content.

(3) A rating of at least four (moderately ill) on the Clinical Global Impression Severity of Illness item (CGI, Clinical Global Impression, 1976).

Patients were excluded if they met DSM-III-R criteria for any other psychiatric disorder coded on Axis I. Suicidal ideation within a year of trial entry, mental retardation, convulsive disorders, alcohol or substance abuse, a history of severe head trauma or suspected organic brain disease, risk of pregnancy, and inability to give informed consent were major exclusion criteria. Conditions likely to interfere with tolerability and efficacy evaluations, such as clinically significant laboratory findings, abnormal electrocardiograms, or an unstable medical disorder were also reason for exclusion. And finally, patients could not enter a trial within 4 weeks of receiving antipsychotic agents in long-acting injectable formulations.

1.2.2 Study Designs

Upon entry into the studies, all psychotropic medications were discontinued during a minimum 2-day washout period (in some studies lasting up to 1 week).

Following the prescribed washout period, patients were randomized to receive drug, placebo, or chlorpromazine according to the study protocol. The maximum dose of quetiapine in the clinical trials varied. In Studies 4 and 8 (low-dose treatment group), the maximum dose was 250 mg daily, while in Studies 6, 7, and 8 (high-dose treatment group), quetiapine-treated patients could be titrated to a maximum of 750 mg daily. Active treatment was titrated upward to the study protocol limit according to the patient's clinical response and tolerability. Therefore, with the exception of Study 4 in which all patients were taken from a dose of 75 mg per day to 250 mg per day in a fixed, stepwise fashion, patients in the other studies were flexibly dosed. There were two additional caveats in the trial designs: doses of quetiapine over 500 mg daily were limited to a duration of 14 days, and treatment with quetiapine was limited to a maximum duration of three weeks in Study 4, and six weeks in Studies 5, 7 and 8.

In establishing the dose of chlorpromazine to be used in Study 7, equivalent clinical antipsychotic potency between quetiapine and chlorpromazine was assumed. Quetiapine and chlorpromazine were then administered in doses up to 750 mg daily. The same dose limitations were applied to chlorpromazine as for quetiapine.

During the studies, patients could be treated for acute agitation and insomnia with chloral hydrate or selected benzodiazepines, depending on the individual study protocol. Extrapyramidal symptoms of at least moderate severity (as assessed by any item on the Simpson Scale (Simpson and Angus, 1970) and of more than 24-hours duration could be treated with benztropine mesylate or an alternative, depending on the study protocol. Diphenhydramine or an alternate could be given for the treatment of akathisia. Provisions were also made to immediately treat acute dystonic reactions, should they occur.

Highlights of the individual study designs are as follows:

Study 4: This was a single-center, 3-week, double-blind, placebo-controlled, parallel-group, rising-dose, pilot efficacy study involving 12 male patients. Unlike later studies, patients entering Study 4 were not required to be acutely psychotic. The entry requirement also called for patients with a BPRS total score of 30 (1–7 point scoring) and 3 (mildly ill) on the CGI-S. Patients in Study 4 were, therefore, less severely ill than those in the multicenter studies that followed.

After a two-day, single-blind, placebo run-in period, patients were randomized to 21 days of double-blind treatment with increasing doses of quetiapine or placebo in a 2:1 ratio. Initially, patients received 25 mg of quetiapine once daily. Doses were increased in increments of 25 to 50 mg approximately every four days until patients reached a final daily dose of 250 mg.

Study 6: After the prescribed minimum two-day placebo phase, patients meeting the entry criteria were randomized to treatment with quetiapine (n=54) or placebo (n=55). Patients on quetiapine were initially given 25 mg three times daily. Thereafter, the doses of drug were titrated upward until an adequate therapeutic effect was achieved. The duration of this and the remaining studies was 42 days, not 21, as in Study 4.

Study 8: Following the minimum two-day drug-free period, patients in this high-dose, low-dose comparison with placebo were randomized to one of three treatment groups: a high-dose regimen of quetiapine (up to 750 mg/day) (n=96); a low-dose regimen of quetiapine (up to 250 mg/day) (n=94); or placebo (n=96). Titrations and limitations were as described in Study 6.

Study 7: In this active comparator study, patients were randomized to quetiapine (n=101) or chlorpromazine (n=100). The dosages were titrated upward as in Studies 6 and 8 according to each patient's clinical response and tolerance for the study drug. The limit for both quetiapine and chlorpromazine was 750 mg per day (not to exceed 500 mg/day for greater than 14 days).

1.2.3 Efficacy Assessments

The severity of each patient's psychiatric symptomatology was rated using several established rating scales. Primary assessments included the 18-item BPRS and the CGI-S in all trials. Secondary assessments varied among trials and included the Modified Scale for the Assessment of Negative Symptoms (Andreason, 1984) (SANS) in Studies 6 and US patients in Study 8 and the negative scale of the Positive and Negative Syndrome Scale (Kay et al., 1987) (PANSS[N]) in Study 7 and the European patients in Study 8.

1.2.3.1 *Statistical Analysis for Efficacy Assessments*

The primary efficacy measures for the placebo-controlled and active-controlled studies were the BPRS total score and the CGI-S. With some exceptions, secondary efficacy measures included the BPRS positive-symptom cluster score (mean of the conceptual disorganization, suspiciousness, hallucinatory behavior, and unusual thought content items), the BPRS negative-cluster symptom score (sum of the emotional withdrawal, motor retardation, and blunted affect items) (only Study 4), the SANS summary score (sum of the global items) and the PANSS(N) total score.

Analyses included patients who were randomized and had at least one post-baseline (on double-blind medication) efficacy assessment (the intent-to-treat population). All assessments were completed just prior to randomization (baseline) and weekly thereafter for the trial durations, unless the patients withdrew from the study before the prescribed end point. In such a case, the assessments were performed at withdrawal and the data carried forward and included in the end point analyses (last observation carried forward or LOCF). The primary analysis was the change from baseline to end point (Study Day 42) for all studies except Study 4, which was Study Day 21.

The change from baseline in BPRS total score, CGI-S score, BPRS positive- and negative-symptom cluster scores, SANS summary score, and PANSS(N) total score were analyzed using an analysis of covariance (ANCOVA) of the change from baseline that included baseline scores (the covariate), center, and treatment in the model. For Study 4, which was a single-center study, center was not included in the model. Statistical significance was defined as a p value of less than or equal to 0.05. Marginal significance was defined as a p value between 0.05 and 0.10. All tests were two-sided.

1.3 DEMOGRAPHY AND WITHDRAWALS

The treatment groups within each trial were generally well balanced with respect to demographic characteristics, including age, gender, race, psychiatric diagnosis, and age at first treatment. With the exceptions noted in section 1.2.2, subjects in the studies were predominantly men in their mid-thirties, who had long-standing illness with multiple hospitalizations; the predominant diagnosis was chronic paranoid schizophrenia. The numbers of patients withdrawing from the studies were similar across studies and study groups. The most common reason for withdrawal from all treatment groups was treatment failure, a typical finding in a population of chronic, moderately to severely ill, hospitalized schizophrenic patients. Mean quetiapine dose and duration of treatment are shown in Table 1.

Table 1. Quetiapine Mean Daily Dose, Duration of Treatment, and Concomitant Therapy

	Quetiapine		Benzodiazepines		EPS Treatment	
Placebo-Controlled Studies						
	Dose±SD (mg/kg)	No Days Mean±SD	n (%)	No Days Mean±SD	n (%)	No D Mean±
Study 4 Quetiapine (n=8)	138±3	21±0	0 (0)	N/A*	0 (0)	N/
PLB (n=4)		18±7	0 (0)		0 (0)	
Study 6 Quetiapine (n=54)	307±134	30±15	17 (31)	7±12	5 (9)	4
PLB (n=55)		27±15	15 (27)	5±5	6 (11)	6
Study 8 (High-dose) (n=96)	360±156	29±15	36 (38)	3±4	7 (7)	8±
(Low-dose) (n=94)	209±42	28±14	48 (51)	5±7	3 (3)	5±
PLB (n=96)		26±15	38 (40)	6±8	10 (10)	4±
Active-Controlled Study						
Study 7 Quetiapine (n=100)	407±124	35±12	40 (40)	16±14	10 (10)	13±
CPZ (n=101)	384±139	33±13	51 (51)	14±13	15 (15)	7±

*N/A = not applicable, SD=standard deviation, PLB=placebo, CPZ=chlorpromazine, EPS=extrapyramidal symptoms

1.4 RESULTS

1.4.1 Overall Efficacy

Overall efficacy was measured in terms of change with respect to baseline for both the BPRS total scores and the CGI-S scores.

Study 4: Baseline scores for the BPRS total score and CGI-S item were similar for both treatment groups. The mean BPRS total scores (Figure 1a) and CGI-cores (Figure 1b) improved steadily from baseline to end point for patients in he quetiapine group. The change from baseline (Study Day 2) in the mean 3PRS total score was significantly greater at Study Day 13 and at end point Study Day 21) for patients who received quetiapine compared with placebo.

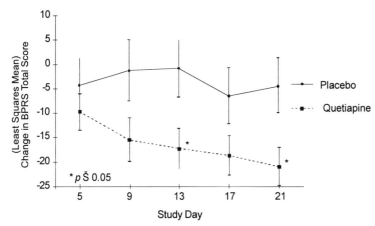

igure 1a Study 4 BPRS mean scores

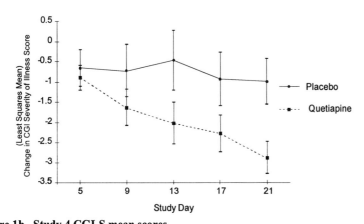

'igure 1b. Study 4 CGI-S mean scores

;tudy 6: The changes from baseline in the mean BPRS total score were ignificantly greater for quetiapine-treated patients than for patients receiving •lacebo at Study Days 14, 28, and 35 (Figure 1c), although at end point (Study)ay 42), the difference between treatment groups was marginally significant.

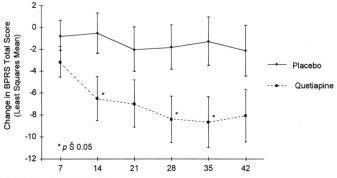

Figure 1c. Study 6 BPRS total scores

Similar results were seen in the CGI-S where the changes from baseline for patients treated with quetiapine were statistically significantly greater than for patients administered placebo at Study Days 21, 28, and 35 (Figure 1d), and were marginally significant at end point.

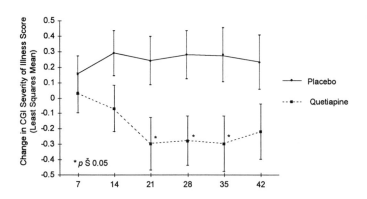

Figure 1d. Study 6 CGI-s scores

Study 8: At most study days, including end point, the high-dose quetiapine group (up to 750 mg/day) showed superior efficacy with respect to placebo for both primary measures of efficacy (see Figure 1e for BPRS total scores and Figures 1f for the CGI-S scores).

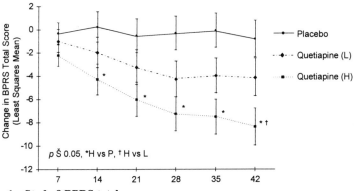

Figure 1e. Study 8 BPRS total scores

High-dose quetiapine was significantly better than low-dose (up to 250 mg/day) quetiapine at end point for the BPRS total score, although the difference for the CGI-S score was marginally significant. The low-dose quetiapine group was not superior to placebo at any time, suggesting that the optimal dose for the treatment of acute schizophrenia is greater than 250 mg per day.

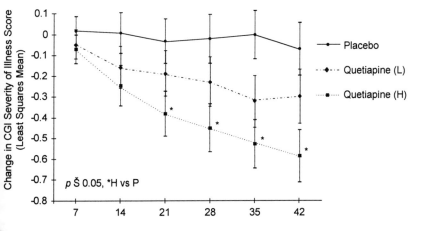

Figure 1f. Study 8 CGI-s scores

Study 7: In the international study comparing quetiapine with chlorpromazine, quetiapine was numerically superior to chlorpromazine on the BPRS total scores and the CGI-S scores (see Figure 2a and b) although there were no significant differences between the two treatment groups at any time point.

Figure 2. Active-Controlled Study: Least-Squares Mean Change from Baseline in the BPRS Total Scores (a) and CGI-Severity of Illness Scores (b) by Study Day (Study 7)

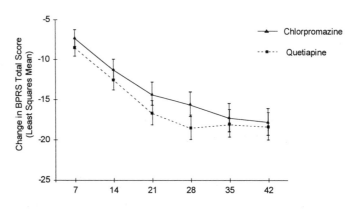

Figure 2a. Study 7 BPRS total scores

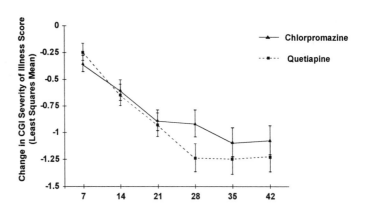

Figure 2b. Study 7 CGI-S scores

Despite this, 65% (64 of 98 patients) of the quetiapine-treated patients exhibited a clinical response to treatment, defined as a decrease from the baseline BPRS total score of 50% or more at any point during randomization, compared with 52% (52 of 98 patients) in the chlorpromazine group, a statistically significant difference.

1.4.2 Efficacy with Respect to Positive Symptoms

Table 2 summarizes the end point results of the positive-symptom cluster scores for the three placebo-controlled studies and the one active comparator study. Individual study results are as follows:

Study 4: Mean BPRS 4-item positive-symptom cluster scores mirrored improvements in the mean BPRS total scores. On the 4-item positive-symptom cluster evaluation, change with respect to baseline favored quetiapine throughout the 21-day study. At end point, the mean change from baseline was -1.0 for quetiapine and essentially 0 for placebo, a significant difference between the treatment groups.

Study 6: Analysis of the BPRS positive-symptom cluster scores showed that significant differences between treatment groups occurred on Study Days 14, 28, and 35. On Study Day 21 and at end point, differences favoring quetiapine were marginally significant for the positive-symptom cluster.

Study 8: Efficacy in the treatment of positive symptoms was corroborated by a statistically significant end point difference between high-dose quetiapine and placebo for change from baseline in BPRS positive-symptom cluster scores. Differences between the high-dose and placebo groups in the mean change from baseline were significant from Study Day 21 onward. At no point were the differences between the low-dose treatment group superior to those for the placebo-treatment group.

Study 7: In the one active comparator study, there were no statistically significant differences between quetiapine and chlorpromazine with respect to the positive-symptom cluster scores.

1.4.3 Efficacy with Respect to Negative Symptom

A summary of the changes from baseline to end point for the BPRS 3-item negative symptom cluster scores, the SANS summary scores and the PANSS(N) total scores for the three placebo-controlled trials and the active comparator trial from the Phase II clinical program are shown in Table 3 (page   ).

Table 2. Mean Change from Baseline at End Point for the BPRS Positive-Symptom Cluster Scores

| | Placebo-Controlled Studies | | | | | | | Active-Controlled Study | |
| | Study 4 | | Study 6 | | Study 8 | | | Study 7 | |
	Quetiapine (n=8)	Placebo (n=4)	Quetiapine (n=53)	Placebo (n=53)	High-Dose Quetiapine (n=94)	Low-Dose Quetiapine (n=92)	Placebo (n=94)	Quetiapine (n=98)	Chlorpromazine (n=98)
Mean (±SD) Baseline Score	2.1 (0.8)	1.9 (0.6)	4.3 (0.9)	4.0 (0.8)	3.6 (1.0)	3.6 (0.9)	3.5 (0.8)	3.8 (0.9)	3.7 (0.9)
Adjusted Mean Change (±SE)	-1.0 (0.2)	0 (0.3)	-0.9 (0.21)	-0.3 (0.21)	-0.9 (0.13)	-0.6 (0.13)	-0.4 (0.13)	-1.7 (0.15)	-1.6 (1.15)
p value*	0.01		0.06		High-Dose v Low-Dose=0.108 High-Dose v Placebo=0.003 Low-Dose v Placebo=0.173			0.72	

* ANCOVA (last observation carried forward),
SD=standard deviation, SE=standard error

Study 4: The mean change from baseline in the BPRS 3-item negative-symptom cluster scores was consistently better throughout the study for patients in the quetiapine—treatment group compared with scores in the placebo—treatment group. These changes were significantly greater at Study Day 15 and at end point.

Study 6: The effects of quetiapine on negative symptoms was demonstrated by statistically significantly greater change from baseline in SANS summary scores in the quetiapine-treated patients, compared with the placebo group from Study Day 21 onward. Patients treated with quetiapine showed improvement in all five of the subscale areas, with the greatest improvement in the avolition-apathy, anhedonia-asociality, and alogia subscales, whereas scores for placebo-treated patients either worsened or did not change.

Study 8: Mean SANS summary scores for patients treated with high-dose quetiapine compared with placebo showed steady improvement from Study Day 7 through end point. The effect of quetiapine on negative symptoms in this trial was less consistent than those observed for positive symptoms. Negative symptoms in US patients were assessed using the SANS summary score while European patients were assessed using the PANSS negative scale total score. Mean SANS summary score in patients treated with high-dose dose quetiapine showed steady improvement from Study Day 7 through end point. Patients treated with low-dose quetiapine had small decreases through Study Day 28, which then increased. Scores for placebo-treated patients increased from Study Day 21 onward, indicating deterioration. Differences in the mean change from baseline in the SANS summary score between the high-dose group and both the low-dose and placebo groups were significant at end point as well as from Study Day 28 onward. Based on the mean changes from baseline for the subscale scores, the high-dose group compared with placebo showed improvement in all five of the SANS subscales.

All three treatment groups demonstrated improvements in negative symptoms at end point as assessed by mean change from baseline in the PANSS(N) total scores. The greatest improvement was in the high-dose group (-4.4) followed by the low-dose group (-2.9). None of the differences between treatment groups, though, was statistically significant.

Study 7: Both treatments were effective in treatment of negative symptoms, measured by reductions in the PANSS(N) total scores. The reductions from baseline were numerically superior in the quetiapine group at Study Days 14, 21, 28, 35, and 42, although the difference between treatment groups was not statistically significant at end point or at any other time point.

Table 3. Mean Change from Baseline at End Point for Negative Symptoms

| | Placebo-Controlled Studies | | | | | | | Active-Controlled Study | |
| | Study 4 (BPRS-neg) | | Study 6 (SANS) | | Study 8 (SANS/PANSS[N]) | | | Study 7 (PANSS[N]) | |
	Quetiapine	Placebo	Quetiapine	Placebo	High-Dose Quetiapine	Low-Dose Quetiapine	Placebo	Quetiapine	Chlorpromazine
	(n=8)	(n=4)	(n=51)	(n=51)	(n=55/38)	(n=51/38)	(n=56/37)	(n=98)	(n=98)
Mean(±SD) Baseline Score	8.9 (1.5)	8.5 (2.6)	14.1 (3.3)	14.0 (3.6)	SANS 15.8 (3.6) PANSS(N) 27.5 (9.4)	SANS 15.8 (3.9) PANSS(N) 25.5 (8.7)	SANS 14.5 (3.6) PANSS(N) 24.4 (6.6)	27.5 (7.6)	27.2 (8.3)
Adjusted Mean Change (±SE)	-5.3 (1.3)	-1.0 (4.1)	-1.0 (0.6)	0.6 (0.6)	SANS -1.7 (0.5) PANSS(N) -4.4 (1.2)	SANS 0.3 (0.5) PANSS(N) -2.9 (1.1)	SANS -0.1 (0.5) PANSS(N) -1.9 (1.1)	-6.6 (0.7)	-6.0 (0.7)
p value*	0.02		0.05		SANS High-Dose v Low-Dose=0.004 High-Dose v Placebo=0.02 Low-Dose v Placebo=0.54 PANSS(N) High-Dose v Low-Dose=0.31 High-Dose v Placebo = 0.10 Low-Dose v Placebo= 0.52			0.5	

* ANCOVA (last observation carried forward), SD=standard deviation, SE=standard error, BPRS-neg=Brief Psychiatric Rating Scale-negative-symptom cluster scores, SANS=Modified Scale for the Assessment of Negative Symptoms Summary Scores, PANSS(N)=Positive and Negative Symptoms Scale-negative scale total scores

2 GENERAL SAFETY AND TOLERABILITY PROFILE

2.1 ASSESSMENTS

Safety and tolerability were assessed by spontaneously elicited adverse events, vital signs, physical examinations, routine clinical laboratory tests including prolactin levels, and electrocardiograms. EPS was assessed weekly using the Simpson Scale. Further evidence for the EPS profile of quetiapine comes from the use of anticholinergic medications to treat EPS and assessments of EPS adverse events (e.g., tremor and akathisia).

2.2 STATISTICAL ANALYSES

All patients who received randomized treatment were included in the analyses of safety and tolerability data. Assessments for adverse events were made throughout the studies for severity and relationship to treatment. Clinical laboratory values, vital signs and weight were summarized using descriptive statistics for actual values as well as for changes from baseline. Change from baseline for plasma prolactin concentrations were analyzed using an analysis of covariance model.

The distribution of the Simpson total scores at baseline was extremely skewed, with the majority of patients having minimum total scores for each scale. Consequently, the use of parametric methods such as ANOVA or ANCOVA was inappropriate for these data. Therefore, frequency distributions of grouped total scores and grouped change from baseline scores were calculated. Changed scores were grouped into categories of improved (change of -1 or less), no change (change of 0), or worsened (change of +1 or greater). The analyses of the grouped change from baseline scores for the Simpson total scores were based on chi-square tests, using Cochran–Mantel–Haenszel methods to control for center effects.

2.3 RESULTS

2.3.1 Overall Safety and Tolerability

Quetiapine was well tolerated in patients treated with the agent during the Phase II clinical trials. The adverse event profiles across these studies were similar (Tables 4 and 5) and most adverse events were rated as mild or moderate. Agitation, somnolence, and headache were the most commonly reported adverse events in the quetiapine—treatment groups. Although the incidence of somnolence was greater for quetiapine-treated patients as compared with patients receiving placebo in the placebo-controlled studies, the incidence of somnolence was similar between treatment groups when quetiapine was compared to chlorpromazine in Study 7. While postural hypotension occurred in a small number of quetiapine-treated patients in the placebo-controlled trials, the incidence of this adverse event in chlorpromazine-treated patients in Study 7 was three times that for quetiapine-treated patients. It is also noteworthy that more than twice as many patients withdrew from the chlorpromazine group compared to the quetiapine group due to an adverse event.

Table 4. Adverse Events Occurring in > 5% of Patients in the Quetiapine and Placebo Groups During Randomized Treatment in the Phase II Placebo-Controlled Studies*

Adverse Events	Quetiapine n=252	Placebo n=155
	n(%)	n(%)
Agitation	70 (28)	33 (21)
Somnolence	67 (27)	18 (12)
Headache	42 (17)	29 (19)
Insomnia	34 (14)	28 (18)
Dizziness	28 (11)	5 (3)
SGPT increased	27 (11)	3 (2)
Constipation	23 (9)	7 (5)
Dry mouth	19 (8)	5 (3)
Tachycardia	18 (7)	7 (5)
SGOT increased	14 (6)	2 (1)
Pain	14 (6)	9 (6)
Infection	10 (4)	10 (7)

*Studies 4, 6, and 8

With respect to clinical laboratory results, quetiapine was associated with mild transient, reversible, and asymptomatic elevations in alanine aminotransferase (ALT) levels in a small subgroup of patients (approximately 5%). These elevations generally resolved despite continued treatment with quetiapine and generally did not exceed five times the upper limits of the normal range of the laboratory assay. Small reductions in mean total T4, and occasionally mean total T3, were observed but were not associated with concomitant elevations in TSH or clinical hypothyroidism. No cases of agranulocytosis were noted.

Table 5. Adverse Events Occurring in > 5% of Patients Treated with Quetiapine or Chlorpromazine During Randomized Treatment in the Phase II Comparator Study

Adverse Event	Quetiapine n=101	Chlorpromazine n=100
	n (%)	n (%)
Somnolence	14 (14)	16 (16)
Insomnia	10 (10)	16 (16)
Dry mouth	8 (8)	6 (6)
Agitation	6 (6)	12 (12)
Anxiety	6 (6)	8 (8)
Hypertonia	6 (6)	3 (3)
Tachycardia	6 (6)	6 (6)
Tremor	6 (6)	3 (3)
Headache	5 (5)	8 (8)
Postural hypotension	5 (5)	18 (18)
Akathisia	4 (4)	6 (6)
Hypotension	3 (3)	7 (7)
Constipation	2 (2)	8 (8)

Quetiapine was not associated with any clinically significant electrocardiogram findings other than a small increase in mean heart rate and occasional sinus tachycardia. Vital signs were similar among the treatment groups in each trial. Clinically significant weight gain, defined as a greater than 7% increase in body weight, was seen in more quetiapine-treated patients than in patients treated with placebo. In Study 6, 24% of the quetiapine-treated patients had a significant weight gain compared with 4% of the placebo group. In Study 8, weight gain appeared to be dose related, as the proportions of patients with clinically significant weight gain were 24%, 15%, and 5% for high-dose, low-dose, and placebo treatment groups, respectively. In the active control study (Study 7), 27% of the quetiapine-treated patients had a significant weight gain compared with 18% in the chlorpromazine treatment group.

2.3.2 Evidence for Atypicality

2.3.2.1 *Prolactin*

Prolactin levels were monitored weekly at most centers throughout the Phase II studies with the exception of Study 4. Prolactin levels decreased in the quetiapine—treatment groups in Studies 6 and 8 and there were no statistically significant differences between the quetiapine—treatment groups and placebo at end point (Hamner, In press; Hong et al., 1995). In the active comparator study, prolactin levels fell in both quetiapine- and chlorpromazine-treated patients with a greater decrease seen in the quetiapine group. At Study Day 42, the difference in mean change from baseline for prolactin between the quetiapine and chlorpromazine groups was statistically significant at end point, favoring quetiapine.

2.3.2.2 *Extrapyramidal Side Effects*

With respect to extrapyramidal side effects in the three Phase II placebo-controlled trials, no statistically significant differences between the quetiapine and placebo—treatment groups were reported in change from baseline for the Simpson Scale grouped scores at endpoint. Overall the results support the conclusion that quetiapine does not induce EPS during short-term administration.

In the Phase II active comparator study, the data demonstrated that both the quetiapine- and chlorpromazine-treated patients experienced few extrapyramidal symptoms as shown by changes from baseline for the Simpson total score. The low level of EPS in the chlorpromazine treatment group was likely due to the use of modest doses (mean dose = 384 mg) during this trial in conjunction with its high intrinsic anticholinergic properties.

Further support for the low EPS liability of quetiapine across the three Phase II placebo—controlled trials includes the similar incidence of EPS adverse events in the quetiapine—treatment groups as compared with the placebo groups (Table 6) and the comparable (and minimal) requirement for anticholinergic agents to treat EPS between the quetiapine and placebo-treated groups (Table 1).

With respect to the active comparator study, there were no withdrawals due to motor systems adverse events in the quetiapine group, whereas one patient in the chlorpromazine group was withdrawn because of an acute dystonic reaction. In addition, the number of patients requiring medications for EPS was slightly higher in the chlorpromazine group than in the quetiapine group (15% v 10% Table1).

Table 6. Summary of EPS Adverse Events* (n[%])

| | Placebo-Controlled Studies | | | | | | | Active-Controlled Study | |
| | Study 4 | | Study 6 | | Study 8 | | | Study 7 | |
	Quetiapine (n=8)	Placebo (n=4)	Quetiapine (n=54)	Placebo (n=55)	High-Dose Quetiapine (n=96)	Low-Dose Quetiapine (n=94)	Placebo (n=96)	Quetiapine (n=101)	Chlorpromazine (n=100)
Total EPS	1 (10)	0	7 (13)	6 (11)	7 (7)	5 (5)	8 (8)	17 (17)	14 (14)
Akathisia	0	0	1 (0)	0	4 (4)	3 (3)	1 (1)	4 (4)	6 (6)
Cogwheel rigidity	0	0	2 (4)	0	0	2 (2)	1 (1)	0	1 (1)
EPS	0	0	1 (2)	1 (2)	1 (1)	0	0	1 (1)	1 (1)
Hypertonia	1 (10)	0	0	3 (5)	1 (1)	0	1 (1)	6 (6)	3 (3)
Neck rigidity	0	0	1 (2)	1 (2)	2 (2)	0	2 (2)	0	0
Tremor	0	0	2 (4)	1 (2)	0	0	5 (5)	6 (6)	3 (3)
Hypokinesia	0	0	0	0	0	1 (1)	0	2 (2)	2 (2)
Akinesia	0	0	0	0	0	0	0	1 (1)	0

*Patients may have had more than one EPS adverse event, EPS=extrapyramidal symptoms

3 PRELIMINARY FINDINGS FROM PHASE III TRIALS

Phase III trials are well underway; two have recently been completed (King e al., In preparation; Arvanitis and Miller., Submitted). Preliminary results a presented at recent international psychiatric association meetings are as follow (Arvanitis, 1995; Fleischhacker et al., 1995):

3.1 MULTIPLE FIXED DOSE, PLACEBO-CONTROLLED TRIAL (STUDY 13)

The primary objective of this double-blind, randomized, multicenter trial was t assess the efficacy and tolerability of quetiapine across a range of fixed doses i comparison with placebo and haloperidol. Inclusion/exclusion criteria wer essentially the same as previously outlined for the Phase II studies in terms o entry scores on the 18-item BPRS total score (≥ 27), the 4-item BPRS positive symptoms cluster (2 of 4 items rated as moderate in severity), and the CGI-S (moderately ill). The patient population was selected from hospitalized patient with acute exacerbation of chronic or subchronic schizophrenia. After a 1 week placebo, single-blind phase, patients were treated for 6 weeks with one of five fixed doses of quetiapine (75, 150, 300, 600, or 750 mg/day), haloperidol (1 mg/day), or placebo. Patients were assessed on randomization and weekly fo efficacy using the BPRS, CGI-S, and SANS. The primary and secondar efficacy measures were the same as previously outlined for the Phase II studie The Simpson Scale was used to assess EPS and TD. Other safety assessment include clinical laboratories, electrocardiograms, vital signs, and physica examinations.

After 6 weeks of treatment, changes from baseline to end point in the mea BPRS total and CGI-S scores showed that quetiapine was superior to placebo fo both primary efficacy measures at end point at doses from 150 to 750 mg/ day with a maximum effect at 300 mg/day. The change from baseline in the BPR total score for the quetiapine 300 mg group was numerically superior to th haloperidol group, although not statistically significantly different. The CGI-S scores for the quetiapine 300 mg and haloperidol—treatment groups wer comparable.

Quetiapine also significantly improved the positive and negative symptoms c schizophrenia. The effects of quetiapine on the positive symptoms were show by improvement in BPRS positive-symptom cluster scores, with mean change from baseline significantly greater for quetiapine-treated patients compared wit placebo-treated patients at doses of 150 to 750 mg/day. The maximum effect wa seen at a dose of 300 mg per day. Changes in SANS summary scores, whic were significantly greater for the quetiapine 300 mg group than for placebo, demonstrated that quetiapine improved negative symptoms.

Overall quetiapine was well tolerated in this study. The rates of patient withdrawals due to adverse events were lower across all quetiapine dose groups than in either control group. The most commonly reported adverse events in the quetiapine treatment groups were headache, agitation, and postural hypotension.

Across all quetiapine dose groups, the incidence of EPS was no greater than that seen in the placebo group, as assessed by grouped Simpson total scores, use of anticholinergic medications, and assessments for EPS adverse events. The quetiapine groups were associated with a lower incidence of EPS compared to the haloperidol treatment group, as assessed by grouped Simpson total score, as well as less frequent use of anticholinergic medication and fewer EPS adverse events. No patients treated with quetiapine were withdrawn because of EPS, compared with four treated with haloperidol and one treated with placebo. Acute dystonic reactions were not observed in the quetiapine—treatment groups.

Similarly, plasma prolactin levels were not elevated in any of the quetiapine dose groups at end point, were substantially lower than those observed for haloperidol, and were not different than those seen in the placebo groups (Hong and Arvanitis, 1995).

3.2 COMPARISON OF DOSE AND DOSE REGIMENS (STUDY 12)

Study 12 was designed to compare the efficacy of quetiapine when administered on twice and three times daily dose regimens. Study 12 was a 6-week, international, multicenter, randomized, parallel group comparison of quetiapine at two different fixed doses (50 and 450 mg/day) and for the latter dose, two different dosing regimens (twice daily and three times daily). Patients were entered into the trial from a pool of hospitalized patients meeting inclusion and exclusion criteria similar to those in the Phase II studies, including a requirement for an acute exacerbation of schizophrenia. The primary measures of efficacy were the BPRS total score, CGI-S, and SANS summary score. Primary measures of tolerability and safety included the Simpson Scale and a battery of clinical laboratories, adverse event assessments, vital signs, and physical examinations.

After a minimum 48—hour washout period, patients were randomized to one of three quetiapine treatment groups (225 mg given in two daily doses, 150 mg given in three daily doses, or 25 mg given in two daily doses). At end point, patients in the 225 mg twice daily group compared to the 25 mg twice daily group, had reduced BPRS total scores, improved CGI-S scores, and reduced

SANS summary scores. The 225 mg twice daily and 150 mg three times daily groups were not distinguishable on BPRS total scores, SANS summary scores, or CGI-S scores. Patients in the 225 mg twice daily dosing group of quetiapine had a similar tolerability profile to the 150 mg three times daily dosing group. No regimen was associated with elevated prolactin. It was concluded from this study that quetiapine can be effectively administered on a twice daily dosing regimen.

These Phase III efficacy and tolerability findings are promising and consistent with previous Phase II results.

4 SUMMARY CLINICAL PROFILE

4.1 EFFICACY

In summary, quetiapine's clinical findings support its designation as an atypical antipsychotic. The results of the Phase II clinical trials have shown it to be superior to placebo and comparable to chlorpromazine in overall measures of efficacy (BPRS total score and CGI-S) in the treatment of hospitalized patients with acute exacerbations of chronic and subchronic schizophrenia. The magnitude of effect was consistent across the trials and in line with those seen in other placebo-controlled trials of antipsychotic agents in development (Beasley et al., 1996; Chouinard et al., 1993). Evidence for quetiapine's efficacy in the treatment of positive symptoms comes from both the placebo-controlled and comparator trials. Positive-symptom cluster scores for the quetiapine treatment groups were consistently superior to placebo and comparable to chlorpromazine and mirrored improvements in the BPRS total scores. With respect to efficacy in the treatment of negative symptoms, quetiapine was superior to placebo as assessed by changes from baseline in the 3-item BPRS negative-symptom cluster in Study 4 and the SANS summary scores in Studies 6 and 8. The reason for the lack of a significant difference between quetiapine and placebo in the PANSS(N) total score in Study 8 is unclear. Regardless of the scale used, severity of baseline negative symptoms appeared to be similar among patients when ratings for subscale global items or PANSS(N) items were reviewed. Differences in the way in which negative symptoms were conceptualized or defined between the two scales may have accounted for some of the discrepancies in the results.

Preliminary findings from the Phase III studies suggest that the effective dose range for quetiapine is 150 to 750 mg per day with the maximal clinical effect for positive and negative symptoms being 300 mg per day. The mean doses used in the flexibly dosed Phase II trials (approximately 300 to 400 mg per day for trial allowing dosing up to 750 mg daily) were consistent with the finding from the Phase III dose ranging study (Study 13). Data from Study 12 also confirmed that quetiapine can be effectively administered on a twice daily regimen.

The efficacy studies from the Phase II and early Phase III clinical studies, therefore, confirm the preclinical findings that suggested quetiapine would be an effective antipsychotic agent with excellent overall efficacy as well as specific efficacy in the treatment of positive and negative symptoms.

4.2 TOLERABILITY

Quetiapine was well tolerated in the clinical trials. The most frequently reported adverse events represented clinical manifestations of schizophrenia (e.g. insomnia and agitation) or were adverse events common to the antipsychotic class of drugs (e.g., somnolence and weight gain). Elevations in liver function tests were observed in a small subset of patients, but none was considered clinically significant and all resolved over time generally with continued dosing of quetiapine. Similarly, decreases in peripheral thyroid hormone levels were noted but they were not associated with elevations in TSH or clinical hypothyroidism. There were no major safety concerns arising from the Phase II trials.

In accordance with the criteria for a low liability for EPS, quetiapine consistently,and across a wide range of doses showed levels of EPS similar to those observed in the placebo groups as measured by the Simpson Scale. The need for anticholinergic medications for treatment-emergent EPS and the duration of their use was also comparable to placebo and lower than for active comparator drugs across the studies. This data further supports the low propensity of quetiapine to induce EPS. A low incidence of EPS adverse events for quetiapine-treated patients across studies also supports the low liability of quetiapine to produce EPS.

Treatment with quetiapine resulted in prolactin levels that were not different from placebo, indicating a favorable endocrine profile compared with standard antipsychotics.

These Phase II and early Phase III studies suggest that quetiapine will be an effective antipsychotic drug and will be associated with low levels of EPS and no sustained elevation in serum prolactin levels. These features are expected to enhance compliance and outcome in the treatment of schizophrenia.

REFERENCES

American Psychiatric Association (1987) <u>Diagnostic and Statistical Manual of Mental Disorders (Third edition, revised)</u>. American Psychiatric Association, Washington, DC.

Andreasen, N. (1984) "Modified scale for the assessment of negative symptoms, NIMH treatment strategies in schizophrenia study". Public Health Administration, Department of Health and Human Services, ADM 9–102.

Arvanitis L. "Seroquel (ICI 204,636), a new 'atypical' antipsychotic: overview of clinical development" (1995) Presented at the 34th Annual Meeting of the American College of Neuropsychopharmacology, San Juan, Puerto Rico.

Arvanitis, L.A., and Miller, B.G. (Submitted) "A multicenter North American comparison of multiple fixed doses of Seroquel™ (quetiapine) in the treatment of patients with chronic schizophrenia".

Barnes TRE. (1989) "A rating scale for drug–induced akathisia", <u>Br. J. Psychiatry</u>, 154, 672–676.

Beasley, C.M., Tollefson, G., Tran, P. et al. (1996) "Olanzapine versus placebo and haloperidol: acute phase results of the North American double–blind olanzapine trial". <u>Neuropsychopharmacology</u> 14, 111–124.

Borison, R.L., Arvanitis, L.A., Miller, B.G. and the US Seroquel Study Group (1996) "ICI 204,636, an atypical antipsychotic: efficacy and safety in a multicenter, placebo–controlled trial in patients with schizophrenia", <u>J. Clin. Psychopharmacol.</u>, 16, 158–169.

Casey, D.E. (1992) "What makes a neuroleptic atypical?" In: <u>Novel Antipsychotic Drugs</u> (Ed. H.Y. Meltzer), Raven Press, New York, pp. 241–251.

CGI, Clinical Global Impression (1976) In: <u>ECDEU Assessment Manual for Psychopharmacology (revised edition)</u> (Ed. W. Guy), United States Department of Health, Education, and Welfare, Rockville, MD.

Chouinard, G., Jones, B., Remington, G. et al. (1993) "A Canadian multicenter placebo–controlled study of fixed doses of risperidone and haloperidol in the treatment of schizophrenia". <u>J. Clin. Psychopharmacol.</u> 13, 25–40.

Fabre, L.F., Arvanitis, L., Pultz, J., Jones, V.M., Malick, J.B. and Slotnick, V.B. (1995) "ICI 204,636, a novel, atypical antipsychotic: early indication of safety and efficacy in patients with chronic and subchronic schizophrenia", <u>Clin. Ther.</u>, 17, 366–378.

Fleischhacker, W.W. and Link, C.G.G. "A multicenter, double–blind, randomised comparison of dose and dose regimen of 'Seroquel' in the treatment of patients with schizophrenia", Presented at the 34th annual meeting of the American College of Neuropsychopharmacology; 1995; San Juan, Puerto Rico.

Gefvert, O., Lindstrom, L.H., Langstrom, B., et al. (1995) "Time course for dopamine and serotonin receptor occupancy in the brain of schizophrenic patients following dosing with 150 mg Seroquel™ TID", Presented at the 34th annual meeting of the American College of Neuropsychopharmacology; San Juan, Puerto Rico.

Hamner, M.B., Arvanitis, L.A., Miller, B.G., Link, C.G.G. and Hong, W.W. (1995) "The effects of Seroquel (ICI 204,636) on plasma prolactin in patients with schizophrenia", Presented at the 50th Annual Meeting of The Society of Biological Psychiatry; Miami. May 20.

Hamner, M.B., Arvanitis, L., Miller, B., Link, C.G.G, and Hong, W.W. (1996) "Plasma prolactin in schizophrenic subjects treated with Seroquel™ (ICI 204,636)", Psychopharmacol. Bull., 32, 107-1100.

Hegarty, J.D., Baldessarini, R.J., Tohen, M., Waternaux, C. and Oepen, G. (1994). "One hundred years of schizophrenia: a meta–analysis of the outcome literature", Am. J. Psychiatry, 151, 1409–1416.

Hong, W.W. and Arvanitis, L.A. (1995) "The atypical profile of Seroquel (ICI 204,636) is supported by the lack of sustained elevation of plasma prolactin in schizophrenic patients". Presented at the 34th annual meeting of the American College of Neuropsychopharmacologists; 1995; San Juan, Puerto Rico.

Kay, S.R., Fisbein, A. and Opler, L.A. (1987). "The positive and negative syndrome scale (PANSS) for schizophrenia", Schizophr. Bull., 13, 261–276.

King, D.J., Link, C.G.G. and Kowalcky, B. (In preparation). "A multicentre, double–blind, randomized comparison of two dose regimens of ICI 204,636 in the treatment of subjects with acute exacerbations of subchronic or chronic schizophrenia".

McGlashan, T.H. (1988). "A selective review of recent North American long–term follow up studies of schizophrenia", Schizophr. Bull., 14, 515–542.

Meltzer, H.Y., Matsubara, S. and Lee, J–C. (1989). "Classification of typical and atypical antipsychotic drugs on the basis of dopamine D–1, D–2 and serotonin–2 pKi values", J. Pharmacol. Exp. Ther., 251, 238–246.

Meltzer, H.Y. (1991) "Dopaminergic and serotonergic mechanisms in the action of clozapine", In: Advances in Neuropsychiatry and Psychopharmacology, Raven Press, New York, pp. 330–340.

Overall, J.E. and Gorham, D.R. (1962) "Brief Psychiatric Rating Scale", Psychol. Rep., 10, 799–812.

Peuskens, J. and Link, C.G.G. (Submitted) "A comparison of ICI 204,636 and chlorpromazine in the treatment of schizophrenia".

Simpson, G.M. and Angus, J.W.S. (1970) "A rating scale for extrapyramidal side effects", <u>Acta Psychiatr. Scand.</u>, 45 (suppl 212), 11–19.

Small, J.G., Hirsch, S.R., Arvanitis, L.A., Miller, B.G., Link, C.G.G. and The Seroquel Study Group (Submitted) "The efficacy and safety of ICI 204,636 (Seroquel) in patients with schizophrenia: a high– and low–dose, double–blind comparison with placebo".

12

PSYCHOSIS IN THE ELDERLY

Raymond J Ancill and Robert J Nielsen

Psychosis in the elderly is common. Between 2% and 4% of the general elderly population has paranoid delusions and 13% of the mentally-impaired elderly are either suspicious or paranoid (Lowenthal, 1964; Blazer and George, in press). However, whether these symptoms represent psychotic illnesses or are nonspecific presentations of neurodegenerative disorders is unclear. Although Kraepelin coined the term "paraphrenia" in 1919 to describe patients who had paranoid delusions but lacked the emotional blunting of those with "dementia praecox" (Kraeplin, 1971), not until 1955 was it realized that for the majority of such patients, the onset of the illness was in the seventh decade of life (Roth, 1955). There is also controversy as to whether or not schizophrenia can emerge in late life, whether geriatric psychosis represents a quite distinct phenomenological entity, or whether paranoid delusions in the elderly are merely the manifestation of organic brain degeneration. These are not idle academic speculations. The use of neuroleptic medications in the elderly is widespread, even in those patients without psychosis, and these drugs are especially toxic in this vulnerable population. A better understanding of the nature of psychotic symptoms in the elderly might, at the very least, identify those patients who might benefit from antipsychotic medications as well as those in whom such treatment would be better avoided.

Perhaps the commonest form of psychosis in old age is that associated with dementia, where it appears that there is a pervasive suspiciousness which leads to memory being accounted for by paranoid or persecutory explanations. This is most evident when an elderly patient claims that a family member or residence manager is coming into their home at night and removing various items such as

Schizophrenia: Breaking Down the Barriers. Edited by S.G. Holliday, R.J. Ancill and G.W. MacEwan. © 1996 John Wiley & Sons Ltd

keys or groceries. The patient is unable to explain why this person is doing this or on what specific evidence they have concluded this. Clearly, the patient has forgotten where these articles were or has failed to purchase the groceries and is compensating for this memory difficulty with pervasive paranoid interpretations. Often there are accompanying auditory hallucinations of a "whispering" type. Unlike the hallucinations of schizophrenia or affective psychoses in younger adults, the auditory hallucinations in the elderly are rarely clear voices saying distinctive words or phrases. More often the elderly patient will state that they can hear people next door or upstairs or in the basement. The voices are muffled or whispering. It is likely that in this case, the patient has a persecutory interpretation of sensory noise due to impairment in hearing. Whether these are, in fact, hallucinations or paranoid delusions is arguable.

However, the most contentious issue in geriatric psychosis is whether or not schizophrenia can emerge in late life. Certainly, the incidence of schizophrenia in the families of persons with an onset of paranoia in later life is increased (Funding, 1961; Rabins et al., 1984). But unlike classic schizophrenia which shows an equal sex incidence, late-onset psychosis demonstrates a preponderance of women (Kay and Roth, 1961; Marneros and Deister, 1984), this increased incidence in women as compared with men having been reported as high as 11:1 (Rabins et al., 1984).

Are there any other differences between early-onset schizophrenia (EOS) and late-onset "schizophrenia" (LOS)? Although cases of LOS demonstrate some familial clustering, the genetic contribution is weaker than has been found in EOS (Rabins et al., 1984). In LOS, there are significantly lower rates of formal thought disorder and the progressive deterioration in personality. This might imply perhaps that there are two distinct but overlapping populations with late-onset psychosis: the first is a form of late-onset schizophrenia but the second is consequent upon organic brain degeneration due to a variety of disorders. Certainly it has been shown that, as mentioned above, impaired hearing is associated with the development of psychotic symptoms in the elderly (Pearlson et al., 1989). It has recently been suggested that atrophy of the planum temporali is associated with the emergence of disordered thought and auditory hallucinations; this area is also involved in hearing and language comprehension. Thus injury to the planum temporali, whether early in life due to neurodevelopmental insults or later in life due to degeneration or ischemia, may alter the function of neuronal areas that involve hearing, language and thought (Rabins, 1994).

Whatever the etiology, the treatment of psychosis, whether in young adults or the elderly, does not depend on putative underlying causes. The use of antipsychotic medication is common in the elderly, even when psychotic features are absent, yet there are few studies indeed to support this widespread use. Furthermore, the elderly are particularly vulnerable to the side-effects of these drugs which themselves can present with the apparent or superficial appearance of a psychosis.

Historically, phenothiazines (especially chlorpromazine and thioridazine) and haloperidol have been widely used in geriatric patients for behavioral control whether there was psychosis or not. The phenothiazines, although powerful tranquilizers, are particularly toxic, with such varied adverse events as postural hypotension, confusion, urinary retention, constipation, acute and tardive dyskinesias, blood dyscrasias, corneal opacities and jaundice. Haloperidol, being a potent but broad-spectrum dopamine blocker, does not have the same wide range of adverse events in the elderly but is very likely to produce disabling dyskinesias, both acute and tardive, even at low doses and even over periods a short as a few weeks. Certainly, when the patient is not even psychotic, potent nonselective dopamine-blocking agents such as haloperidol are best avoided, especially as haloperidol is not particularly tranquilizing. Loxapine is another neuroleptic that has been used quite widely, at least in Canada, for psychosis and for dysfunctional, aggressive behavior in the demented elderly. Although it is not an ideal drug, there is evidence to suggest it is significantly better tolerated than haloperidol in the elderly, especially in the area of extrapyramidal side-effects (Carlyle et al., 1993). More recently, risperidone has been introduced as a selective antipsychotic agent blocking D2 and 5-HT2 receptors. This has the net result of making risperidone a serotonergic antipsychotic by virtue of the fact that it blocks the postsynaptic serotonin "off-switch", thus allowing serotonin levels to rise while blocking D2 receptors selectively. There are, however, to date no published studies of the use of risperidone in the elderly.

A retrospective review of clinical experience of the use of risperidone in elderly patients with psychotic symptoms was carried out. Eighteen consecutive cases were identified by reviewing the inpatient and outpatient records of the Geriatric Psychiatry Program at St. Vincent's Hospital, Vancouver. There were 14 females and 4 males. The average age was 73, ranging from 63 to 85 years.

Diagnoses were as follows:

Affective psychosis	11	(61%)
Dementia with psychosis	3	(17%)
Parkinson's disease with emergent psychosis	3	(17%)
Schizophrenia	1	(5%)

Of the 18 cases, 9 (50%) had failed to tolerate a previous neuroleptic (see Table 1). Initial doses of risperidone were 0.5 mg h.s. in 5 cases, and 0.5 mg h.s. b.i.d. in the remaining 13. Where there had been significant neuroleptic toxicity in the past, 0.5 mg h.s. was chosen.

Table 1

Neuroleptic Discontinued	Reason for Discontinuation
Loxapine	Delirium (one months duration)
Loxapine	Extrapyramidal side effects (EPS) and increased cognitive impairment.
Loxapine	EPS
Perphenazine	EPS
Haloperidol	Tardive dyskinesia
Thioridazine	Visual disturbance
	FINAL DOSE
Methotrimeprazine	Over sedation
Methotrimeprazine	EPS
Stelazine	EPS

Of the 18 patients on risperidone, only one patient was discontinued and this was due to a rise in creatinine kinase which was otherwise asymptomatic. The patient was still on the initial dose of 0.5 mg b.i.d. and had shown no improvement. Final doses are detailed in Figure 1, with the commonest dose being 1 mg per day (56%). No other treatment-emergent side-effects were noted. The remaining 17 patients were rated on a Clinician's Global Impression as 'moderately improved' or better. Two patients (11%) were rated as "moderately improved", 13 patients (72%) were rated as "much improved" and 2 (11%) were assessed as "very much improved".

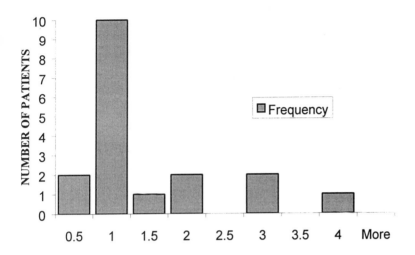

Figure 1. Risperidone Case Series: Final Dosage Levels

It would, therefore, appear that risperidone is both effective and well tolerated in this particularly vulnerable population. Furthermore, this patient group, although retrospective and part of an open case series, were consecutive patients for whom risperidone was indicated and prescribed and showed the significant female preponderance of psychosis in the elderly (3.5 to 1). The lack of emergent toxicity is important as 50% of the patients treated with risperidone had failed to tolerate a previous neuroleptic. This benign profile may represent both an intrinsic lower incidence of side-effects with risperidone as well as careful use of low doses, significantly lower than those suggested for younger adults.

REFERENCES

Blazer D, George LK, Hughes D. (in press) "Schizophrenic symptoms in an elderly community". In <u>Epidemiology of Aging</u> (eds. J. Brody and Maddox G.L.), Springer, New York.

Carlyle W., Ancill R.J., and Sheldon L.J. (1993). "Aggression in the demented patient: a double-blind study of loxapine versus haloperidol", *International Clinical Psychopharmacology*, 103-108.

Funding T. (1961). "Genetics of paranoid psychoses in later life", *Acta Psychiatrica Scandinavica*, 37:267-282.

Kay D.W.K., and Roth M. (1961). "Environmental and hereditary factors in the schizophrenias of old age ("late paraphrenia") and their bearing on the general problem of causation in schizophrenia", *Journal of Mental Science*, 107:649-686.

Kraepelin E. (1971)(original 1919). *Dementia Praecox and Paraphrenia*, translated by Barclay R.M. (eds Robertson G.M., Huntington N.Y., and Kreiger R.E.).

Lowenthal M.F. (1964). *Lives in Distress*, New York, Basic Books.

Marneros A. and Deister A. (1984). "The psychopathology of "late schizophrenia". *Psychopathology*, 17:264-274.

Pearlson G., Kreger L., and Rabins P.V. (1989). "A chart review of late-onset schizophrenia", *American Journal of Psychiatry*, 146:1568-1574.

Rabins P.V. (1994). "Implications of late-life onset schizophrenia: a new hypothesis".
In *Schizophrenia: Exploring the Spectrum of Psychosis* (eds Ancill R.J., Holliday S. and Higenbottam J.), John Wiley & Sons, Chichester.

Rabins P.V., Pauker S., Thomas J. (1984). "Can schizophrenia begin after age 44?", *Comprehensive Psychiatry*, 25:290-293.

Roth M (1955). "The natural history of mental disorder in old age", *Journal of Mental Science*, 101:281-301.

Index

Note: Page references in *italics* refer to Figures; those in **bold** refer to Tables

Index compiled by Annette Musker